EMERGENCY:

A Guide for Ambulance Personnel

ABOUT THE AUTHORS

Mike Walsh has a wealth of practical experience gained as a Charge Nurse in the A&E Department of Bristol Royal Infirmary. Whilst there he wrote his very successful book *Accident and Emergency Nursing* and made a full-length BBC TV documentary on the work of the Accident Service. He now lectures at Bristol Polytechnic, specialising in this field.

Tom Eddolls is a qualified Ambulanceman on Emergency duties. He has been a member of the Avon Ambulance Service for nine years, eight of them spent on front line duties in Bristol. He is Extended Trained, with the Drugs Therapy Certificate and is a Registered Member of the Association of Emergency Medical Technicians. He holds the NHS Training Authority's National, Extended Ambulance Aid Certificate and in 1986 he won the 'Fred Townsend Memorial Award' in its inaugural year.

EMERGENCY:

A Guide for Ambulance Personnel

Mike Walsh BA SRN PGCE
Lecturer in Nursing, Bristol Polytechnic

Tom Eddolls REMT
Ambulanceman, Avon Ambulance Service

Heinemann Professional Publishing

Contents

Appendices

1. Resuscitation

INTRODUCTION

Anyone can save a life. That is the positive starting point for this book. Of course there will be many situations when life cannot be saved, but there are also many other occasions where the combination of certain skills and a cool head can literally be lifesaving. In this first chapter we look at the basics of resuscitation: simple principles and practical steps that combined can preserve a life which would otherwise be lost. Whether readers are National Health Service workers or part of a voluntary ambulance crew, first aiders, service medics or whatever, they can save a life. In order to simplify the text, the term *paramedic* will be used throughout to cover these and all other emergency personnel who may be in a position to render such vital assistance.

BASIC RESUSCITATION

We need to start by asking the obvious question: how do we know when resuscitation is needed? This opens up a general principle of fundamental importance for all emergency work: start by assessing the situation quickly but carefully. The old adage about look before you leap is very apt in emergency work; it is only when you have assessed your patient to form some idea of the principal problems, and put them in some order of priority, that you can begin your work. Without proper assessment much of what you do may be irrelevant or even harmful to the patient, while essential care may be overlooked altogether.

We need to have, therefore, a simple scheme of assessment with an order of priority relevant to the patient's crucial needs. Such a scheme is referred to as the *ABC* of resuscitation: A for airway, B for breathing and C for circulation (it is worth including cervical spine as well as circulation under C, but more of this below).

Airway

When you are called out to collapsed patients the first step is to check their airway (Fig 1.1). Is it clear or obstructed? If the

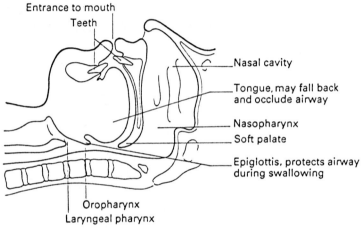

Fig. 1.1 The upper airway

airway is not clear, insufficient oxygen will reach the lungs and no amount of effort will resuscitate the patient. Commonly encountered obstructions include vomit, blood or other inhaled material such as food or dentures. Trauma to the upper respiratory tract or neck may cause the airway to be blocked by swelling around the trachea or windpipe – for example, inhalation of flames, steam or hot gases or a severe blow to the neck. Even an insect sting can produce such severe swelling as to block the airway. If patients are unconscious and lying on their back, the tongue can flop backwards and block the airway very easily.

Causes of Obstructed Airway

In assessing the airway, the paramedic should check for evidence of breathing: Is the chest wall moving up and down? Can you hear breathing if you place your ear to the person's mouth? If not, then either the airway is completely blocked, or the patient has stopped breathing for some other reason. If the airway is partly blocked the breathing will be very noisy and laboured. The alert paramedic will often be able to spot vital clues such as evidence of vomit or blood around the nose and mouth, while inspection of the patient's mouth may reveal the actual cause of the blockage. A pen torch is most useful, but great caution should be exercised in using a laryngoscope in this situation (see below).

The other likely cause of an obstructed airway is the tongue flopping backwards if the person is unconscious and lying on his/her back. Budassi and Barber (1984) recommend the head tilt–jaw lift manoeuvre as the most effective way of clearing the airway (Fig. 1.2). This involves tilting the head back and lifting

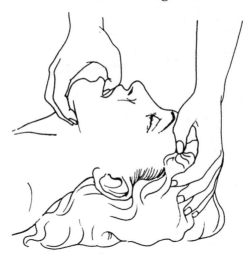

Fig. 1.2   Head tilt–jaw lift manoeuvre. The mandible is pulled forward using the thumb and forefingers

the chin forwards far enough to almost close the mouth. However, caution is vital, as if the patient has sustained a cervical spine injury, the paramedic could cause disastrous harm to the spinal cord in this way. Simons and Howell (1986) point out that tilting the head by lifting the neck could be disastrous for an injured neck. It is therefore recommended that if cervical spine injury is suspected, as an alternative measure the head should be kept still in a neutral position and the jaw pushed forward using fingers and thumbs, minimising neck movement (Fig. 1.3).

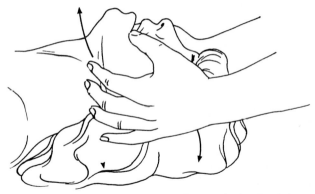

Fig. 1.3   Jaw thrust manoeuvre for cervical spine injury

Either way the tongue will be lifted away from the posterior pharynx and the airway opened.

If the paramedic has established that the patient's airway is obstructed by some foreign material then every effort should be made to clear it as quickly as possible, using fingers if necessary. Always remove false teeth. If suction equipment is available this should be used with a rigid wide-bore suction catheter of the Yankaur type; flexible, narrow suction catheters are of little use in an emergency situation if the patient is vomiting semidigested food.

Maintaining a Clear Airway

When the airway is cleared a most valuable aid to maintaining it is the oropharyngeal airway (Guedel, for example; Fig. 1.4). It should be introduced via the side of the mouth in an upside-down position, and then rotated and slid over the back of the tongue, keeping the airway clear. However, if patients cough and gag on the airway then they are sufficiently conscious to protect their airway themselves, so the oropharyngeal airway may be withdrawn.

The next step required to maintain a cleared airway is to roll patients onto their side into what is known as the recovery position (Fig. 1.5). This will mean that if the patient vomits or if there is bleeding into the mouth, the fluid will tend to drain readily out of the side of the mouth rather than be inhaled. This position should be combined with the head tilt–chin lift position to ensure a good clear airway which may then be protected with

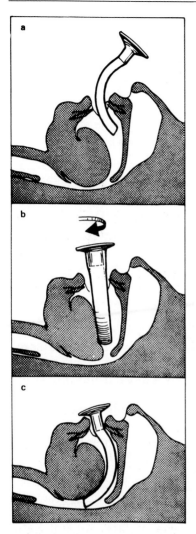

Fig. 1.4   Guedel airway insertion

an oropharyngeal airway if the patients can tolerate it. A word of caution here: before moving patients, always ask yourself if there is any risk of a cervical injury. If so, they should only be moved in accordance with the log-rolling technique outlined on page 55 as serious spinal cord injury may otherwise result.

By following the simple principles of clearing any obvious obstructions, and then preserving the airway by a combination of positioning and the use of an oropharyngeal airway, you will have taken the first big step in keeping your patient alive.

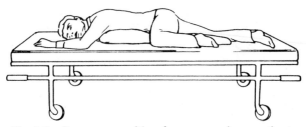

Fig. 1.5 Recovery position for unconscious patients

Breathing

The first obvious question here is whether the patient is breathing at all.

A further sign of severe breathing difficulties is the presence of *cyanosis*, where the patient appears to be a blue-grey colour in the face, especially around the lips, which means that it can be seen in those of African/Asian origins as well as in Caucasians (white-skinned persons). It may also be noticed at the finger ends and in the toes and feet – the extremities of the circulation.

Listen: look closely at the chest wall, remove clothing if you have to, check the rate of breathing, is it very shallow or of normal depth? Is the chest expanding equally and at the same time on both sides (failure to do so indicates serious chest trauma; p. 60)? To make sure you know what normal breathing looks like find a suitable volunteer and observe.

Breathing is such an essential part of everyday life that it is taken for granted, yet you will only recognise abnormal breathing when you know what the norm is. How much does the chest normally move up and down and at what rate? Find out for yourself with the aid of your volunteer!

Mouth-to-mouth Resuscitation

Cyanosis is a late sign of severe respiratory failure, and therefore an indication that urgent action is needed.

If no breathing at all is discernible, then the paramedic must use mouth-to-mouth or expired air resuscitation at once. The best position for this is to lie patients flat on their back and use the head tilt–chin lift position to ensure a clear airway. Place your mouth over the patient's and pinch the nostrils shut to prevent air escaping through them. In this position, having taken a deep breath first yourself, breathe out inflating the patient's lungs as you do so, and you should see the chest wall rise slowly. Fisher (1986) recommends starting resuscitation with two rapid breaths in quick succession. After this initial spurt, try to keep a rate of one breath every 5 s. If there is severe trauma to the mouth, it may be possible to breathe through the patient's nose, keeping his or her mouth sealed as much as possible. In young children both mouth and nose may be enclosed by the rescuer's mouth, though it must be remembered that young children have a much smaller lung capacity, so smaller, more frequent breaths are required.

The Heimlich manoeuvre

If no movement of the chest wall is seen, either the seal between your mouth and the patient's is not tight enough, there is a deep obstruction to the airway, or you are not blowing hard enough. One method of clearing an obstruction, such as a piece of partly chewed food accidentally inhaled, is the Heimlich manoeuvre (Fig. 1.6). This should be used if the simple method of hitting the

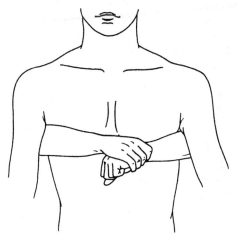

Fig. 1.6   Heimlich manoeuvre for standing patient

person several times in the small of the back is not possible or has been tried and has failed. If patients are flat on the floor, face up, straddle them and apply your hands to a point midway between the umbilicus and the tip of the sternum (breastbone). With the heels of your hands apply a firm pressure both inwards and upwards, repeating this several times. The aim is to try to expel the offending object from the part of the respiratory system that it is blocking by increasing the pressure (with a sudden sharp push) within the intrathoracic (chest) cavity. If patients are choking on food in this way and still standing, then the manoeuvre may be carried out by standing behind them and grasping your arms around them to meet in front at the same point, then pulling them back towards you suddenly, driving your clenched fists inwards and upwards to achieve the same result (see Fig. 1.6).

Exhaled air contains nearly as much oxygen as inhaled air, therefore mouth-to-mouth respiration is capable of supplying sufficient oxygen to patients to allow for recovery, provided that oxygen reaches the lungs. Even greater amounts of oxygen may be delivered to patients at far less effort to the paramedic by use of an oxygen cylinder and bag/mask system; this is considered later in the chapter (p. 17).

Circulation

Is the patient able to pump enough oxygenated blood around his or her body? Each beat of the heart will pump about 70 ml of blood into the main circulation via the aorta and a similar volume to the lungs, while with exertion this amount may double (Green, 1978). This surge of blood into the circulation produces the familiar pulse which is readily felt at the wrist in the radial artery. If you can feel a pulse there you need to note its rate and rhythm.

The *rate* is the number of beats per minute and can be estimated by counting over a 30 s period and multiplying by two. The *rhythm* is also important as it should be regular with each pulse of the same strength, so if there is irregular rhythm or varying strength, urgency is indicated.

Absence of Pulse

If patients are unresponsive do not waste time looking for the radial pulse, but try to find the carotid pulse in the neck instead (Fig. 1.7). This is located much nearer the heart so if patients have a pulse at all, this is where it can be felt. Absence of the carotid pulse indicates that the heart has no effective output and patients are in a state of cardiac arrest. Make sure you can locate this pulse immediately (in other words practise finding it on your friendly volunteer!). It is the absence of a carotid pulse in collapsed unresponsive patients that indicates the need for urgent action.

Irreversible brain damage will occur within 2–3 min of cardiac arrest (Green, 1978) unless intervention occurs. However, Baskett and Zorab (1977) point out that patients who appear to have

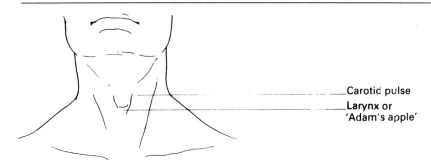

Fig. 1.7   Location of carotid pulse

arrested may still have had a minimal cardiac output which was undetectable, so it is therefore worth commencing resuscitation if the time from collapse is a little longer than the 3 min quoted above. Immediate intervention is required, with no time to wait for help to arrive – resuscitation *must* start at once in the absence of a carotid pulse. Other signs which may be present include cyanosis and dilated pupils, but these usually develop after cardiac output has ceased, so do not bother to wait for them as they are late signs.

Chest Compression

With chest compression the aim is to imitate the heart's pumping action and attempt to pump blood around the body. The basic requirements are that patients should be flat on their back on a hard surface – if they have collapsed sitting in a chair, for example, or on a bed, they must be moved quickly onto the floor. Kneel beside them, place the heel of one hand two fingers' width from the base of the sternum, and then place the other hand over the first hand (Fig. 1.8). The aim is then to compress the chest by giving steady, downward thrusts onto the sternum with about half your own body weight, arms straight, using a rocking motion. Always ensure that your hands are in contact with the sternum as there is a risk of fracturing ribs if you inadvertently press away from it. The aim should be to compress the sternum in an average adult 4–5 cm (1½–2 in) (Budassi and Barber, 1984), thereby expelling blood from the heart and large vessels of the chest around the body. The blood, however, must be oxygenated, and that requires expired air or mouth-to-mouth resuscitation, as described on page 6. As one cannot do cardiac compression at the same time as mouth-to-mouth respiration, it is recommended that a rhythm of 15 compressions to 2 breaths is

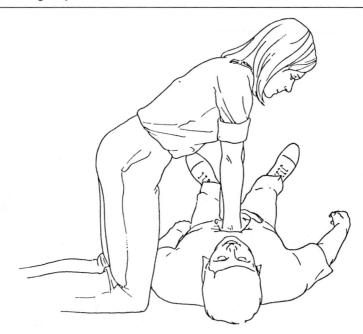

Fig. 1.8   Position for chest compression

established, with the aim of trying to compress the chest 80 times/min, giving 15 breaths in the process (Fisher, 1986).

If working single-handed, this will soon become very tiring, but persevere in your efforts for as long as possible. This tiring procedure underlines the importance of trying to raise the alarm immediately. If you have an assistant, you need to establish a clear pattern of compressions to each breath, say 5:1.

With a child the rate of compression needs to be quicker, 80–100/min depending on the age of the child (the younger the child, the quicker the rate). Similarly, the force used in compressing the sternum needs to be less: use one hand for a child, or two fingers of the hand in the case of a baby, aiming for a compression of 1.5–4 cm (½–1½ in) depending on the child's age.

Always remember to check that the airway is clear before you start. While you are working on the patient, stop occasionally to feel for a carotid pulse to see if you have been successful. The golden rule is *do not give up*, even if it is half an hour before help comes.

By attending to the basic ABC of resuscitation as described above, a supply of oxygenated blood can be maintained to the vital parts of the body until either recovery occurs spontaneously or more sophisticated help arrives on the scene. Even then the three basic principles of ABC still apply.

ADVANCED RESUSCITATION

What we have described above can be applied by anyone who finds themselves at the scene of a collapse, whether in the street, home, workplace or outdoors. However, it is possible to improve considerably the patient's chances of recovery with the use of certain equipment, provided that the paramedic has been well trained in its use, has a grasp of the key principles involved, and follows at all times the basic ABC framework and local policy guidelines.

Advanced Equipment

Let us first of all consider the patient's airway. Great emphasis has been placed on clearing it, and suction equipment is invaluable for this (see Appendix B, Fig. B.7). Portable suction pumps are now available, working off a small battery-driven motor. Always ensure before going on duty that the battery has been properly charged, the motor is working and you have a selection of different suction catheters from the narrow, long flexible type to the rigid wide-bore Yankaur variety.

Suction Catheter

In a Yankaur suction catheter (see Appendix B, Fig. B.7) you will find a small hole where your hand would grip the catheter. As long as this hole is open, no suction is applied at the tip of the catheter, as the suction force will be through the hole. Close it with your thumb and you then have suction at the tip. The best technique is to introduce the catheter as far as you can with the hole open (and therefore no suction at the tip), then withdraw it with the hole occluded by your thumb, which gives suction at the business end of the catheter as you withdraw. Wide-bore, rigid catheters are designed for oral use, while the long flexible catheters are best used to suck out an endotracheal tube.

Laryngoscope

This piece of equipment will allow you to see clearly what is happening at the back of the patient's pharynx (Fig. 1.9 and Appen-

EQUIPMENT

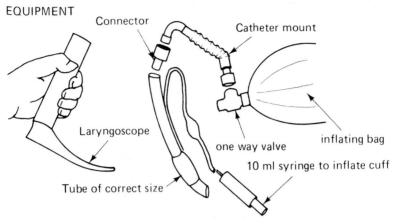

Connector

Catheter mount

Laryngoscope

one way valve

inflating bag

Tube of correct size

10 ml syringe to inflate cuff

Always check
(i) That the equipment fits together
(ii) That the laryngoscope works

Tube sizes
8·0 mm for almost all adults
6·0 mm for 8 - 12 year olds
4·0 mm for 3 - 7 year olds

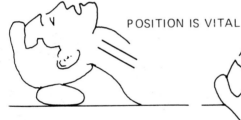

POSITION IS VITAL

Correct position
Flex neck and extend head on neck;
this straightens the route to the larynx

Incorrect position
Extending the neck
makes things more difficult

LANDMARKS

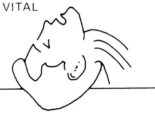

Teeth

Mandible

Tongue

Palate

Uvula

Epiglottis

Larynx and trachea

Oesophagus

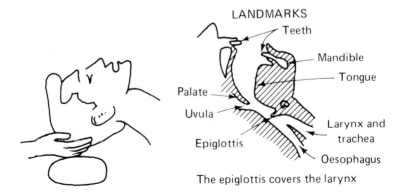

The epiglottis covers the larynx

INTRODUCING THE LARYNGOSCOPE

Hold laryngoscope in <u>left</u> hand

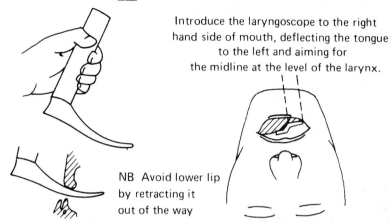

Introduce the laryngoscope to the right
hand side of mouth, deflecting the tongue
to the left and aiming for
the midline at the level of the larynx.

NB Avoid lower lip
by retracting it
out of the way

THE POSITION OF THE LARYNGOSCOPE

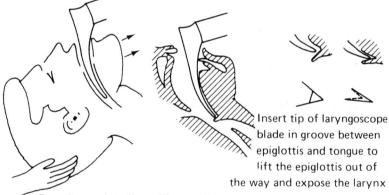

Insert tip of laryngoscope
blade in groove between
epiglottis and tongue to
lift the epiglottis out of
the way and expose the larynx

Draw larynx into line with mouth by
upward and forward lifting of laryngoscope in line with the handle

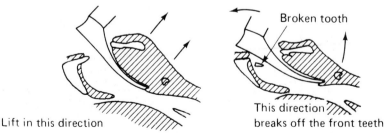

Broken tooth

Lift in this direction

This direction
breaks off the front teeth

Fig. 1.9   The laryngoscope (from Easton, 1977)

dix B, Fig B.9). It consists of a blade that slides over the back of the tongue, allowing it to be moved out of the way, and a light to illuminate the area being investigated. With a laryngoscope, an excellent view may be obtained of the oral cavity down as far as the epiglottis. Apart from being an essential tool for intubation of the patient (see below, p. 15), the laryngoscope allows close inspection of the mouth and airway with excellent lighting. Foreign bodies may then be seen and removed more readily (a pair of Magill's forceps (see Appendix B, Fig. B.9) are a vital adjunct to a good suction catheter) and sources of bleeding can be more easily identified. *Caution*: a laryngoscope should not be used in the case of an ill child with a history of drooling and difficulty in breathing, as this could be epiglottitis and the blade could provoke a fatal laryngeal spasm.

Both suction equipment and laryngoscope should be thoroughly checked before going on duty: check the batteries, is the bulb working and tightly screwed in place? Have you got spares in case you break a bulb accidentally?

Oropharyngeal Airway

Correct positioning of the head has already been described as a means of keeping the airway clear in unconscious patients, while the use of an oropharyngeal airway (such as Guedel; see Fig. 1.4) will keep the tongue from flopping backwards to block the airway. Inhalation of vomit or blood can lead to severe lung damage (aspiration pneumonia) or even asphyxiation, so a more secure method of maintaining the airway is desirable if there is facial trauma and bleeding or a high risk of vomiting.

Intubation

In order to secure the airway on a more permanent basis an endotracheal tube (ET) may be introduced with the aid of a laryngoscope, a procedure known as intubation. As can be seen from Fig. 1.9 (and Appendix B, Fig. B.9) an endotracheal tube is basically a plastic tube, long enough to be introduced via the mouth into the trachea. It has an inflatable cuff which when blown up provides a seal so that no vomit or blood should be able to find its way down into the lungs. Disposable endotracheal tubes are available in a variety of sizes, 8 mm being suitable for most adults, 6 mm for 8–12-year-olds and 4 mm for 3–7-year-olds.

Baskett and Zorab (1977) have pointed out that with cardiac arrest or deeply unconscious patients intubation is the ideal method for securing the airway, especially if there is a high risk of aspiration of blood or vomit, for example.

Correct Positioning

The first step in intubation, after checking again that all your equipment is in working order and that suction is ready and running, is to get the head and neck in the correct position; with patients flat on their back, flex the neck forward and extend the head back, but do not extend the neck as this makes matters more difficult. A pillow under the neck will be a great help in positioning.

Introduce the laryngoscope blade just to the right of the midline and, following the natural curves of the mouth, slide it over and behind the tongue. You can now lift the tongue upwards and forwards with the blade in the midline and the tongue displaced to the left side of the mouth; but resist the temptation to lever the blade against the front teeth to bring the tongue forward, as you may dislodge any loose teeth with disastrous results for the patient's airway which at this stage is not protected (this is why you need your suction available and running). The handle of the laryngoscope should be at a 45° angle to the horizontal at this stage (see Fig. 1.9).

As you place the laryngoscope blade into the space between the base of the tongue and the epiglottis, you will see the glottic opening into which we are aiming to introduce the endotracheal tube. The laryngoscope should be held in the left hand and the endotracheal tube in the right, so it can be slid from the right side of the mouth through the glottic opening into the trachea. The cuff should be inflated immediately with 5–10 ml of air from a syringe.

It now remains to check that the tube is in the correct place, as it may possibly be in the oesophagus. If air is blown into the tube, the chest wall should expand equally. If the abdomen rather than the chest wall is seen to inflate, the tube is in the wrong place—possibly due to the length of the tube; it may have been introduced via the trachea into the right main bronchus, the effect of this is that no air will be blown into the left lung. Listen with a stethoscope to both sides of the chest, and if all is well you should hear air entering into both lungs. If in doubt, Budassi and Barber (1984) advise pulling back slightly on the tube which should allow ventilation of both left and right bronchus and lung. Endotracheal tubes are very generous in length, so Baskett and Zorab therefore advise measuring the distance from the corner of the mouth to the ear; double this and you have the correct length for the tube. If it is too long and time allows you can shorten it with scissors.

Advantages of Intubation

These are as follows:

(1) It provides control of the airway.
(2) Your patient is protected from the risk of aspiration.
(3) Suctioning of the trachea is now possible (using an aseptic technique).
(4) There is less risk of gastric distension due to blowing air into the stomach (this is always a risk when using an oropharyngeal airway or no airway at all, as may be the case if you happen upon a situation off-duty).
(5) It does not interfere with chest compression.
(6) Intermittent positive pressure ventilation (IPPV) with up to 100% oxygen delivered by a bag and connector system, or mechanical oxygen resuscitator and connector system, is possible (see p. 17 and Figs. B.8 and B.13).

Intubation Technique

Intubation is a skilled technique that can only be learnt by actually doing it. Fortunately dummies are available for practice, but there is no substitute for the real thing. Fortunately in many areas schemes are now being set up with local hospitals to allow paramedics to obtain experience with a skilled anaesthetist, intubating patients routinely prior to surgery. Once learnt, like any practical skill, practice is crucial to achieve a high standard of performance, so every opportunity should be taken to practise this vital skill when hospital-based refresher courses are available.

A point to remember is that during insertion patients are not being ventilated nor are they receiving any chest compression (although once inserted a tube does not interfere with compression). Make sure they are well oxygenated before insertion therefore, and if you fail at the first attempt withdraw the tube and make sure the patients receive some oxygen and chest compression before trying again.

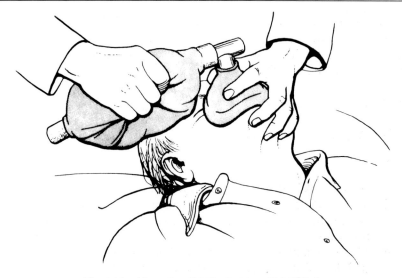

Fig 1.10   Use of self-inflating bag and mask

Bag and Mask System

A bag and oxygen system may be used to improve considerably the efficiency with which the patient's lungs are ventilated (Fig. 1.10 and Appendix B, Fig. B.8). Various companies market bag and mask systems, the common elements of which are:

(1) A compressible bag which acts as a reservoir for oxygen and, when squeezed by hand, will deliver sufficient volume to inflate both lungs;

(2) Connecting tubing to attach the bag to a supply of oxygen, usually a cylinder for ambulance use;

(3) A detachable mask, various sizes being available to ensure a tight fit with the patient's face;

(4) An attachment that fits onto an endotracheal tube (see Appendix B, Fig. B.9);

(5) An escape valve that prevents exhaled air mixing with incoming oxygen.

The bag can either be used with a mask to ventilate patients who have an oropharyngeal airway *in situ* or, with the mask removed, it may be connected to an endotracheal tube to allow easy ventilation of the patient's lungs with a high concentration of oxygen.

Transtracheal Catheter Ventilation

If the obstruction to the airway is so severe that intubation is not possible—for example, there is a foreign body that cannot be removed—then a rapid alternative means of gaining access to the airway is needed. Budassi and Barber (1984) advise transtracheal catheter ventilation as a means of achieving this.

The point we are looking for is the cricothyroid membrane which can be felt by placing a finger on the Adam's apple and then moving down 3 cm. If possible the skin should be wiped with an alcohol swab to reduce infection risks. The widest-bore intravenous cannula available should be used, attached to a syringe. The cannula should be advanced firmly but gently through the skin and cartilage underneath, while gently pulling back on the syringe to apply a negative pressure. When the cannula reaches the trachea, air will enter the syringe. Remove the metal stylette to leave the cannula in the trachea, then after removing the syringe, connect up the end of the cannula to an intravenous giving set, the other end of which can be attached to an oxygen cylinder. If there is spontaneous breathing, it will be necessary to disconnect the tubing from the cylinder each time the patient breathes out as there is no escape valve in this system. If there is no spontaneous breathing, use the pressure of the oxygen in the cylinder to inflate the lungs, disconnect the tubing from the cylinder and the chest wall will be seen to fall as exhalation occurs by passive recoil. Minimum pressure only must be used, just enough to inflate the lungs as shown by a rise in the chest wall. Such a system can provide the patient with sufficient oxygen until hospital is reached.

CARDIAC MONITORING

Figure 1.11 is a simple diagram of the heart and, as can be seen, the two large, lower chambers of the heart do most of the work. The right ventricle pumps blood to the lungs where it is enriched with oxygen, and the left ventricle pumps this oxygen-rich blood to the rest of the body.

The beating of a person's heart is in response to minute electrical currents that are conducted along specific pathways, thus stimulating the muscles surrounding the four chambers of the

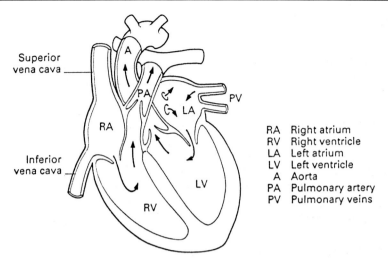

Fig. 1.11   Diagram of the heart; arrows indicate direction of blood flow

heart to contract and pump blood around the body. The regular and efficient beating of the heart is essential for health and life. Monitoring the electrical activity of the heart may therefore yield vital information about the patient's condition which will in turn enable emergency personnel to render more effective care in the crucial prehospital stage.

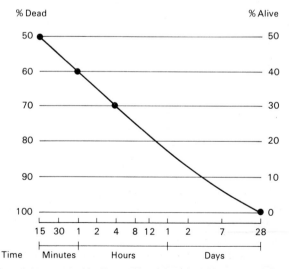

Fig. 1.12   Cumulative fatality against time in 348 coronary heart attacks where death occurred within 28 days (adapted from Tunstall Pedoe, 1978)

Just how critical this stage is may be demonstrated by considering the work of Tunstall Pedoe (1978). In a study of persons dying from heart attacks he found that 60% of deaths occurred within 1 h of the attack, when the patient is most likely to be in the care of ambulance crew rather than in hospital (Fig. 1.12).

Electrocardiography

Monitoring the electrical activity of the heart is known as electrocardiography, and the resultant electrocardiograph, be it displayed on a monitor screen or recorded on paper, is known as an ECG (see Appendix B, Fig. B.11). It contains vital information, correct interpretation of which could be lifesaving.

The point to remember is that the ECG is simply a picture of the heart's electrical activity, recorded with the aid of very sensitive electrodes that are attached to the chest wall in the pattern shown in Fig. 1.13. In the accident and emergency department a

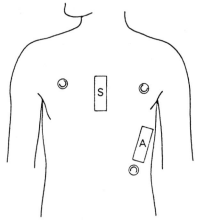

Fig. 1.13   Location of electrodes for three lead ECG monitoring and paddles for defibrillation (S=sternum, A=apex)

more detailed ECG may be performed using leads attached to the feet and wrists as well as in six different chest positions. This is known as a twelve-lead ECG and reveals a great deal of detailed information that can assist the medical staff in their management of the patient. However, for monitoring the patient in order to detect life-threatening changes in rhythm the three chest leads will suffice. Changes from the normal rhythm are called arrhythmias, and it is these life-threatening arrhythmias that the paramedic should be able to detect.

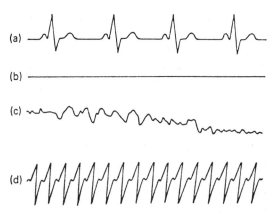

Fig. 1.14   Some ECG readings: (1) normal sinus rhythm; (b) asystole; (c) ventricular fibrillation; (d) ventricular tachycardia

Rhythms and Arrhythmias

Figure 1.14 illustrates the normal rhythm, or sinus rhythm (as it lies in the sinoatrial node or pacemaker of the heart). It also shows the three most urgent arrhythmias, asystole, ventricular fibrillation and ventricular tachycardia. *Caution*: look at your *patient* at all times, for it is the patient you are treating not the ECG monitor! Simple faults, such as an electrode that is loose or has fallen off, or vibration from the vehicle if you are moving quickly, can look very like these arrhythmias and lead to disastrously wrong conclusions if you do not check your patient's clinical condition. Asystole is the absence of cardiac activity, while ventricular fibrillation will not produce any significant output from the heart. Either way, if your monitor is correct, no blood is circulating. Therefore, if your patient is sitting upright holding a conversation with you then a monitor showing asystole is incorrect. Always interpret the monitor according to the patient's clinical condition.

Asystole is a state of cardiac arrest. Ventricular fibrillation means that the bundles of muscle fibres in the ventricles are not beating together in the normal coordinated fashion that pumps blood around the body, merely twitching independently of each other, so there is no output from the heart, and the result is effectively cardiac arrest. A further condition that may arise is known as electromechanical dissociation: here the ECG will look normal as the heart's electrical activity is still functioning; however, it is failing to produce any muscular contraction of the myocardium so again there is no cardiac output. This underlines the importance of looking after the patient and not the ECG monitor—you could have a normal trace on the monitor, yet the patient would be in a state of effective cardiac arrest. In all these cases, resuscitation should start at once.

Ventricular tachycardia, with a rate of around 180 beats/min may spontaneously revert to a normal rhythm but it can progress to fibrillation and arrest. On the other hand the patient may have a very slow rate (say, 20–40 beats/min); this is known as bradycardia, and leads to a lack of oxygenated blood reaching the vital centres of the body.

Defibrillation

For patients who are in a state of cardiac arrest, further vital interventions can increase their chances of survival. Passing a direct current shock through the heart while it is in a state of ventricular fibrillation may be sufficient to knock it back into a normal rhythm. This intervention is only effective in ventricular fibrillation, not asystole, and is therefore known as defibrillation. It appears to work by depolarising (discharging the electrical energy stored within) the cells of the myocardium, thereby terminating the chaotic electrical activity responsible for fibrillation. Having wiped the slate clean it is possible then for normal electrical impulses transmitted through the conducting pathways to take over and start up a normal heart rhythm.

Note: Ventricular fibrillation can be coarse or fine.

Defibrillators

Defibrillators (see Appendix B, Fig. B.11) are usually powered by rechargeable batteries, and can be preset to deliver the required charge (measured in joules, J). Older machines are calibrated in stored energy while more modern ones use delivered energy (as in this text); thus 400 J stored is the equivalent of 320 J delivered, and 200 J stored the equivalent of 160 J delivered.

The two paddles can, on most machines, be used as ECG electrodes to monitor the heart rhythm between shocks. A conducting medium should be used to maximise the effectiveness of the shock and prevent skin burns. Although electrode gel can be used, specially made pads are preferable. Many different types of defibrillators are available, so it is important that the crew know their model well. A cardiac arrest allows no time to consult the manufacturer's instruction handbook!

Defibrillating sequence

The following general sequence is suggested for undertaking defibrillation:

(1) Check that there is no ECG monitor error: are electrodes in place? Is the patient's clinical condition consistent with diagnosis, that is, no carotid pulse, collapsed condition?

(2) Expose the chest.

(3) Apply defibrillator pads to chest.

(4) Switch defibrillator on.

(5) Charge to 160 joules (J).

(6) Place paddles in correct positions (see Fig. 1.13) ensuring that nobody is touching either ambulance trolley or patient, or else they too will receive the shock.

(7) Press the trigger, observing a twitch of the body as the shock is given.

(8) Feel the carotid pulse, check monitor for rhythm.

(9) If pulse is felt, administer oxygen via mask and monitor condition closely as further episodes may occur. Keep checking the pulse as well as the ECG monitor.

(10) If no pulse is felt, give 15 chest compressions, check the ECG and if still in ventricular fibrillation deliver 160 J shock. Repeat as necessary, delivering 320 J for subsequent shocks.

Baskett and Zorab (1977) point out that if the heart muscle (myocardium) is poor in oxygen, this will make defibrillation much less likely to be successful in starting the patient's heart working again. Maximum oxygenation during the period before defibrillation should therefore increase the chances of success.

DRUGS DURING RESUSCITATION

The patient's chances of survival can be greatly improved if certain key drugs can be given during resuscitation. There is still controversy surrounding the subject of ambulance personnel giving such powerful drugs in the field, and each health authority has its own policy which should be strictly adhered to. However, Vincent (1986), in reviewing advanced training for ambulance crew in Brighton, considers their use of drug therapy to have been safe. The principal drugs used in resuscitation are as follows (see Appendix B, Fig. B.12).

Lignocaine

If the patient is in coarse ventricular fibrillation and three shocks have failed to restore a normal rhythm with output, an intravenous injection of 100 mg lignocaine can be given before the fourth shock, as it acts by suppressing the excitability of the heart muscle.

Lignocaine may also be used to control ventricular tachycardia, when 100 mg (10 ml of 1% solution) should be given slowly over at least a 2 min period intravenously, but only if there is a palpable pulse. Solutions of lignocaine 0.1 % in glucose injection are available in 500 ml packs for continuous infusion (1 mg of lignocaine per 1 ml of glucose 5 % solution). If ventricular tachycardia persists after the initial injection of lignocaine and the patient remains conscious with a palpable pulse then i.v. lignocaine should be given at the rate of 4 mg/min for 30 min, dropping to 2 mg/min for the next 2 h (*British National Formulary (BNF)* 1984). (If the patient showing ventricular tachycardia is collapsed and pulseless, then synchronised cardioversion with the defibrillator is needed to shock the heart back into a normal rhythm. The shock must be timed to avoid the T wave as, if fired at the same time, it may lead to ventricular fibrillation. The defibrillator should have a synchronised shock control which may be activated to deliver the shock at the correct time to avoid this risk.)

Lignocaine can also be used to suppress multiple ventricular ectopics. If these are occurring frequently (say, more than every fourth beat) and the systolic blood pressure is less than 80, then the heart is in a dangerous condition. An i.v. injection (100 mg) should therefore be given slowly over several minutes.

Adrenaline

This powerful drug is capable of stimulating the myocardium. Where the arrhythmia is still fine ventricular fibrillation, following three defibrillation attempts, 5 ml of 1:10 000 adrenaline should be given before attempting the fourth. If the patient is in asystole, 5 ml of 1:10 000 solution should be given intravenously as it will help electrical discharge from the two key nodes of the heart's conducting system, atrioventricular and sinoatrial (Camm, 1986). Adrenaline should also be given if there is electromechanical dissociation.

Note: A second 5 ml can be given in each case if necessary.

Atropine

The parasympathetic branch of the autonomic nervous system has many effects, one of which is to act as a 'brake' on the heart, and stop it going too fast. However, sometimes its effect can be detrimental to the patient, for instance when the heart rate drops to only 30–40 beats/min. Atropine can block this effect and speed up the heart to a more effective rate. So if the patient has a rate below 50 and a systolic blood pressure below 70, then atropine 0.5 mg i.v. (this dose can be repeated once) will improve the circulation. With asystole or electromechanical dissociation, an i.v. injection of 1 mg atropine should be given immediately before the adrenaline injection to counteract this braking effect.

Sodium Bicarbonate

Once the heart stops pushing a normal circulation around the body, various complex chemical changes will occur; one of the principal effects is to make the blood more acid than normal, making it harder to restart the heart. It is therefore essential to give an intravenous alkaline solution to neutralise this extra acidity and return the blood chemistry to normal. The standard solution used is sodium bicarbonate 8.4%, which comes in units of 50 ml (pre-packed syringe) or 200 ml (polyfusor). Insert a venflon, then administer 50 ml after 15 min from the time of arrest and a further 50 ml after another 15 min if resuscitation is continuing. Then flush the venflon through with 5 ml of Hepsal, or another solution such as normal saline may be run in slowly, simply to keep the intravenous line patent for administration of other drugs as needed. The principles involved in setting up intravenous infusions (i.v.i.s) are discussed below (p. 35).

Note that lignocaine, atropine and adrenaline may be given via the endotracheal tube (ET) where they will be absorbed through the lining of the lung. Even if an i.v. line has not been immediately established, these drugs can still be given, although in twice the dosage. Remember that this does not apply to sodium bicarbonate which can only be given intravenously. If local policy permits, drugs such as these can be given after myocardial infarction (see p. 24) in order to stabilise the patient's heart prior to transfer to hospital. Appropriate drug therapy may well prevent cardiac arrest.

SUMMARY OF ADVANCED CARDIOPULMONARY RESUSCITATION

A summary of advanced cardiopulmonary resuscitation is shown in Table 1.1.

Table 1.1   Advanced cardiopulmonary resuscitation

Monitor ECG

Ventricular fibrillation	*Asystole*
Defibrillate 160 J	Atropine 1 mg i.v.
Defibrillate 160 J	Adrenaline 10 ml/1:10 000 i.v.
Defibrillate 320 J	Sodium bicarbonate 50 ml/8.4%

If coarse VF:
Lignocaine 100 mg i.v.
Defibrillate 320 J

If fine VF:
Adrenaline 5 ml/1:10 000 i.v.
Defibrillate 320 J

Sodium bicarbonate 50 ml/ 8.4% i.v.
Defibrillate 320 J

Note: Drug doses given are for a 70 kg adult. Child doses should be scaled down on a proportional weight basis.

Chest compression and ventilation should be maintained as long as no pulse is felt. If the asystolic patient develops ventricular fibrillation, treat accordingly. Note that the energy levels stated here are delivered not stored energy (corresponding to 200 J and 400 J, respectively).

In this introductory chapter we have seen how basic, simple steps can help resuscitate a critically ill patient. With the addition of extra equipment and training, plus the use of certain drugs and defibrillation, you and your ambulance crew can improve the patient's chances of survival dramatically, providing that at all times you keep your cool and stick to the basic principles outlined in this chapter. Whatever happens, keep cool and don't panic: your patient's life may not depend so much on how much you know, but on how you apply it!

References

Baskett P., Zorab J. (1977) Essentials of emergency management. In Easton K. (ed.) *Rescue and Emergency Care.* London: Heinemann (Out of print).

British National Formulary (1984) London: BMA and The Pharmaceutical Society of Great Britain.

Budassi S., Barber J. (1984) *Emergency Care.* St Louis: C. V. Mosby Co.

Camm A. J. (1986) Asystole and electromechanical dissociation. In Evans T. R. (ed.) *ABC of Resuscitation,* London: *British Medical Journal.*

Easton, K. (ed.) (1977) *Rescue and Emergency Care.* London: Heinemann. (Out of print).

Fisher J. M. (1986) Recognizing a cardiac arrest. In Evans T. R. (ed.) *ABC of Resuscitation.* London: *British Medical Journal.*

Green J. H. (1978) *An Introduction to Human Physiology.* Oxford: Oxford Medical Publications.

Macleod J. (1984) *Davidson's Principles and Practice of Medicine.* Edinburgh: Churchill Livingstone.

Simons R., Howells H. (1986) *The Airway at Risk.* In Evans T. R. (ed.) *ABC of Resuscitation.* London: *British Medical Journal.*

Tunstall Pedoe, H. (1978) The Tower Hamlets Study. *British Heart Journal,* **40**: 510.

Vincent R. (1986) Resuscitation by Ambulance Crews. In Evans T. R. (ed.) *ABC of Resuscitation.* London: *British Medical Journal.*

Walsh M. (1985) *Accident and Emergency Nursing, A New Approach.* London: Heinemann.

2. Shock

INTRODUCTION

Shock is a term often used very loosely. In this chapter it will be used specifically as it relates to the patient's circulation. Walsh (1985) describes the condition as: insufficient oxygen reaching the tissues of the body which if not corrected quickly will cause a series of complex physiological changes that will eventually

Table 2.1 Classification of Shock by Cause

Type of Shock	Cause
(1) Hypovolaemic	
Haemorrhagic	Blood loss due to soft tissue bleeding, fractures, wounds
Burns	Loss of plasma in burn exudate
Dehydration	Major body fluid loss, such as vomiting, diarrhoea, diabetes and other metabolic disorders
(2) Cardiogenic	Failure of heart as pump leading to inadequate circulating blood volume, for example, after heart attack
(3) Vasogenic	
Septic	Endotoxins from bacteria can cause massive dilatation of circulation in certain severe infections
Anaphylactic	Severe allergic reaction: histamines cause dilatation of capillaries and arterioles. Can be rapidly fatal and needs urgent attention

become irreversible and lead to the patient's death. Shock may therefore be thought of as a failure of the circulation, for whatever reason, to transport enough oxygen to the tissues of the body. The three main types of shock—hypovolaemic, cardiogenic and vasogenic are summarised in Table 2.1.

As can be seen from Table 2.1 there are a variety of ways in which the patient can develop shock, varying from major injury to serious illness. The steps needed to prevent shock from developing into a fatal condition vary with the type of shock, so careful assessment of the situation is mandatory.

SIGNS OF SHOCK

The failure of the circulation to move sufficient oxygenated blood around the body reveals itself in several ways that the paramedic must be able to recognise in order to diagnose shock. The three classic signs are: air hunger; drop in blood pressure; and speeding up of respiratory and pulse rates. In air hunger, to try to compensate for circulatory failure the patient's body attempts to increase its intake of oxygen by increasing the depth and rate of respiration. At rest a normal respiratory rate is somewhere between 12 and 16 breaths per minute, but in shock this may be increased. However, there are many other reasons why a patient may breathe faster, such as pain or anxiety, so on its own a rapid respiratory rate does not indicate shock.

Systolic and Diastolic Blood Pressure

The falling volume of blood circulating around the body will cause a drop in blood pressure, another classic sign of shock. Blood pressure is measured as two readings, systolic and diastolic. *Systolic* blood pressure is that generated by the heart each time it beats, and *diastolic* pressure is the resting pressure between beats. Blood pressure (BP) is measured in millimetres of mercury (mmHg), and is written with systolic pressure first, then diastolic. Green (1978) states that a typical blood pressure for an average young adult is around 120/80; this tends to increase with age so that for a person of, say, 65 a blood pressure of 150/90 is a normal recording. In dealing with shock, the crucial measurement is the systolic pressure, and shock develops if that falls below 90.

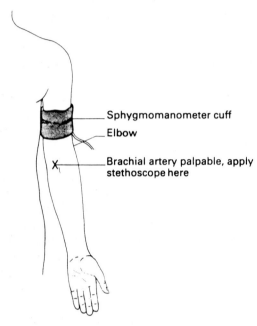

Fig. 2.1   Location of brachial pulse (used for taking blood pressure)

Recording Blood Pressure

In order to record blood pressure both a sphygmomanometer and stethoscope are needed. The cuff of the sphygmomanometer is wrapped around the patient's arm just above the elbow (Fig. 2.1). The next step is to locate the brachial pulse, and once this has been found the end of the stethoscope should be placed over this point and the cuff inflated to significantly above the likely blood pressure. The pressure in the cuff should then be gradually reduced by means of the attached valve. When the pressure has been reduced to just equal to the systolic, the heart will now be able to force blood back into the brachial artery past the cuff, and this can be heard with the stethoscope as a gentle tapping sound. As the pressure in the cuff is reduced to the diastolic pressure the sound changes in nature and becomes muffled before fading out altogether. This muffling of sound is taken as the diastolic pressure. (An alternative convention takes the fading out of sound as the diastolic pressure, so be sure you know which convention is used in your authority.) Recording blood pressure is not easy at first, and requires practice to get accustomed to the sounds for which one is listening. Once mastered though it becomes second nature, and the information gained from an accurate reading of your patient's blood pressure is well worth the trouble taken in obtaining it.

Caution: in using a low systolic blood pressure (less than 90) as the basis for diagnosing shock, a word of warning. The body has a series of compensating mechanisms which can raise blood pressure for a short period of time, despite heavy bleeding. It would be unwise, therefore, in dealing with an injured person whose blood pressure is 120/80, to think that there is no danger of shock. Compensation involves closing down the circulation to the periphery, hence the patient's skin will appear cold, clammy and pale, a sign that should always alert you to the danger of shock developing, even if blood pressure appears normal.

If the blood pressure falls, the body attempts to compensate by asking the heart to beat faster. Thus it is usual to find that in the development of shock as the blood pressure falls so the heart rate speeds up. This is the third classic sign of shock, a speeding up of respiratory and pulse rates coupled with a falling blood pressure.

Hypovolaemic Shock

In dealing with hypovolaemic shock caused by trauma, the evidence of volume loss is usually visible to the paramedic. Budassi and Barber (1984) suggest that the loss of 15% of circulating blood volume will lead to the development of shock, while at 30% severe hypovolaemic shock will develop. For the average adult of 70 kg (about 11 stone) this translates to about 0.75 litres and 1.5 litres respectively (about 1⅓ pints and 2⅔ pints). Estimating the volume of blood spilt from a wound is notoriously difficult, but it is essential to do this (Fig. 2.2). Try to think of a pint bottle of milk: if an average-sized person has lost much more than that, they will begin to develop shock. The accident and emergency staff will appreciate any estimate you can give them of the amount of blood lost on site; this is vital information.

Volume loss may not be as easily measured as visible bleeding. This applies in burn cases, in particular. Settle (1974) suggests

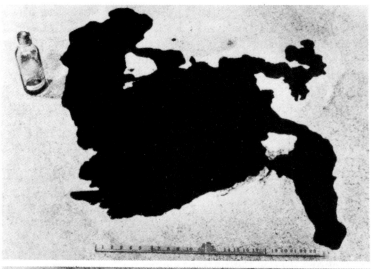

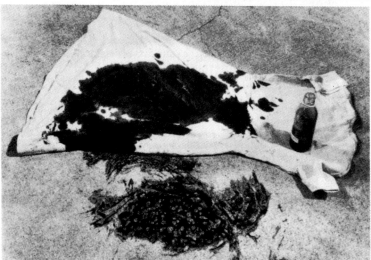

Fig. 2.2   Bloodshed: (a) one donation on an unabsorbent surface makes a pool about 60 cm (2 ft) square; (b) half a donation will soak a dress right through and leave a considerable amount of blood on the surface beneath it. (Reproduced by kind permission of Camera Talks Ltd from the film strip *How much blood?*)

that if the significantly burnt area exceeds 15% of body area, then shock will develop due to plasma loss from the burnt tissue. Alternatively, bleeding may be internal and therefore not readily visible. For example, the blood loss from a fracture of the femur is around 1 litre, while fractures of the pelvis may cause blood loss of up to 2 litres.

Evidence of volume loss, characteristic changes in the vital signs and the appearance of cold, pale and clammy skin are vital clues for emergency personnel in diagnosing shock. Finally, the patient may start to become drowsy and confused. Settle (1974) describes loss of consciousness as indicating approaching death (Table 2.2).

Table 2.2   Summary of Signs of Shock

---

(1) Rapid breathing, development of air hunger
(2) Rapid pulse, thready in nature when felt
(3) Falling blood pressure, systolic below 90
(4) Visible evidence of blood loss over 0.5 litres (1 pint)
(5) History suggestive of serious injury or illness
(6) Pale, cold, clammy skin
Late signs
(7) Drowsiness
(8) Loss of consciousness

BASIC PRINCIPLES OF TREATMENT

The immediate treatment of shock will depend upon the cause, but some basic principles are fairly universal. First, as the root cause of the problem is a lack of circulating oxygen in the body, oxygen should always be administered via a high concentration face mask, say 4 litres/min (see page 116 for the exception to this rule, i.e. the patient who suffers from long-term respiratory illness). The failing circulation can be aided by increasing venous return to the heart (Green, 1978), which may be effected by elevating the legs to improve the drainage of venous blood from the lower limbs. The patient is probably best laid flat while this is done. Pain, may exacerbate shock, so every attempt should be made to relieve it, together with anxiety and fear.

If the shock is hypovolaemic in nature—this is probably the most common sort encountered—then an obvious specific intervention is to try to control blood loss. With an open wound this is best done by direct pressure to the actual wound itself. Fountain and Westaby (1985) describe this as the simplest and best method of controlling bleeding, and state that 5–10 min firm pressure will be sufficient to stop the bleeding in most cases, even in large wounds. *The use of tourniquets is unnecessary, often harmful and potentially very dangerous, and should be actively discouraged.* Direct pressure with a bulky dressing will control bleeding from even the severest of wounds, including amputations, bleeding will be further lessened by elevating the injured part, so that blood loss from even the worst combat or high energy road traffic wound can be stemmed without recourse to tourniquet (Beverly and Coombs, 1985).

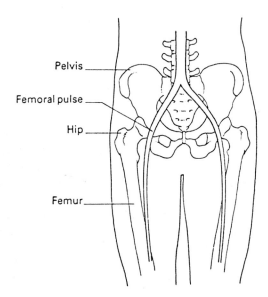

Fig. 2.3   Location of femoral pulse

The use of pressure points to stem bleeding is rarely needed except perhaps to allow a clear view of the wound in a bloodless field. Such pressure should only be applied for a few minutes at the very most as serious damage can occur if the limb is starved of blood for any length of time. Both brachial and femoral artery are conveniently used for this purpose (Fig. 2.3).

In dealing with shock due to burns, clearly it is not possible to stop the loss of fluid from an extensive area by direct pressure. The reader is referred to Chapter 5 for a full discussion of the burnt patient. The basic principles of giving oxygen, pain relief and improving venous return to the heart still apply.

Before considering replacement therapy, we should consider other forms of shock where i.v. fluid replacement is unnecessary. In cardiogenic shock the problem is not one of a lack of circulating volume, but rather of failure of the pump (the heart), so this should not be treated with fluid replacement, but the other basic principles still apply. In anaphylactic shock the extreme allergic reaction (for example, to drugs such as penicillin, or bee stings, etc.) is at the root of the problem, with the result that after the initial ABC of resuscitation has been considered, drugs should be administered: adrenaline (0.5 mg–1 mg, i.m., repeated if needed); an antihistamine such as chlorpheniramine (10–20 mg, i.m. or slowly i.v.); and hydrocortisone (100–500 mg i.m. or slowly i.v.), not large volumes of i.v. fluids.

INTRAVENOUS INFUSION TECHNIQUE

As stated above, for many forms of shock the replacement of lost fluids is the key to successful treatment. By the time patients have reached a hospital facility, their circulation may have collapsed so much that resuscitation is impossible, or precious time may be wasted trying to find a vein to site a drip.

Given that the best chance of successfully starting a drip is when the paramedic finds the victim rather than later when they reach hospital, and that the sooner fluid replacement begins the better it is for the patient, there is now a widespread recognition of the need for paramedics to be able to set up intravenous infusions (i.v.i.s, see Appendix B, Fig. B.10).

Inevitably there will be variations depending on local policy, but the following section outlines the basic principles.

Finding and Gaining Access to the Vein

The first step is to gain access to the vein that is to be used for the intravenous infusion. The paramedic has to make the choice, usually a large superficial vein in the arm, to make siting easier, and also to accommodate the large volume of fluid that may need to be infused. Coco (1980) points out that the most obvious veins may not be the best as they have a tendency to roll, that is move under the skin when one attempts to cannulate them; she recommends anchoring the vein with the thumb during cannulation as a precaution against this. Jointed areas should be avoided if possible as movement of the joint by the patient (such as bending the elbow) may dislodge the cannula or at the least greatly slow down the flow of fluid. Figure 2.4 shows some of the principal superficial veins of the arm suitable for i.v. sites, which the paramedic needs to be able to identify immediately in an emergency situation.

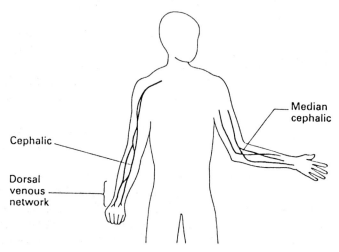

Fig. 2.4   Common sites for intravenous infusions. The median cephalic vein on the inside of the elbow (antecubital fossa) is used for emergencies as it is large and offers easy access. However it is close to the brachial artery and being situated at a joint suffers from the disadvantage that joint movement will impede the intravenous infusion. The cephalic vein or dorsal venous network is therefore preferred for cases where large volumes of intravenous fluid are not needed, or for the siting of a heparinised venflon with intravenous infusion attached

Intravenous Cannulation

In order to facilitate cannulation of the vein, the i.v. cannula usually contains a steel needle, the aim being to use the needle to gain access to the vein, then withdraw it leaving the plastic cannula in the vein. The following procedure is suggested:

(1) Run the drip through the giving set that you are going to use. It is no use having a cannula in the vein if you have nothing to connect it to! (See p. 37 for details of giving sets.)

(2) Apply a tourniquet to make the veins more prominent (for example, blood pressure cuff inflated to between diastolic and systolic pressure).

(3) Hang the arm below the level of body, as this helps veins to fill if patient is in a collapsed condition; allow up to 1 min for filling.

(4) Select a vein and swab site with antiseptic if possible.

(5) Hold the arm straight and explain to patient what is to happen and why.

(6) Place the needle with the bevel on the needle end facing upwards just below where you intend to enter the vein.

(7) Enter the skin no more than 6.25 mm (¼ in) from where you intend to enter the vein, using firm but gentle pressure. Keep the angle between the needle and the skin to a *maximum* of 45°.

(8) Move upwards through the tissue towards the vein, reducing the angle the needle makes with the skin, until it is nearly parallel with the skin.

(9) Pick up the vein and slide the needle in, being careful not to go through the vein and out the other side. There should be a back flow of blood indicating successful entry. Move cautiously about 6.25 mm (¼ in) up the vein and withdraw the needle about 12.5 mm (½ in). Then insert the venflon fully.

(10) Secure cannula with tape.

(11) Connect to the i.v. giving set and release the tourniquet.

(12) Check that i.v. fluid flows freely.

(13) Secure the cannula in the vein with a firm adhesive dressing and splint the arm if a site over a joint was used.

If you have not been successful in locating a vein, withdraw the needle immediately as unnecessary trauma and pain can be caused. Apply firm pressure over the site for 4 min (the patient or a passerby can do this) to prevent bleeding and bruising, and try elsewhere with a fresh i.v. cannula. *Do not use* the same cannula as it will have become contaminated.

Caution: It is important to handle used needles very carefully as there is always the risk that the patient may be suffering from a disease such as AIDS or hepatitis that can be transmitted via blood. Even the most minor accidental needlestick injury with a used needle should be reported for your own safety.

Mention has been made of the need to run the drip through

before cannulating the vein. An i.v. giving set consists of sterile plastic tubing with a connector at one end to fit onto the i.v. cannula, and a spike at the other which allows it to be introduced into the bag of i.v. fluid. In between there is a drip chamber which allows flow rate to be measured, and a roller clamp that controls the rate.

Fluid Containers

Intravenous fluids are held in different sorts of containers. The two sorts that will most concern paramedics are either a soft plastic bag that collapses gradually as fluid runs out of it, and a semirigid plastic container known as a *polyfusor*. Two forces push the i.v. fluid through the giving set into the patient. The first is atmospheric pressure which, due to the soft nature of the container walls, will gradually collapse the container as fluid runs out. Second, note that the system operates by gravity feed, therefore the i.v. fluid needs to be above the level of the patient's heart at all times. Any kinks in the giving set will prevent a free flow of fluid, while if the drip is sited near a joint such as the elbow, bending of the joint will interfere with the infusion. When an intravenous infusion has been set up it is important to note the times and types of fluids that have been given for the benefit of the medical staff at the accident and emergency unit.

Solutions

It now remains to consider the different types of fluids that are available and the situations in which they are given. In dealing with a hypovolaemic patient it will be remembered that the main problem is a dangerous loss of fluid from the circulation. Ideally this would be replaced with blood, but as blood has to be stored under very specific conditions of temperature, and must be exactly cross-matched to make sure the patient gets the right group, this is not a practical solution. A fluid used a great deal to replace lost circulating volume is called *Haemaccel* (gelatin) a synthetic substance that can be retained in the circulation because of its large molecular size. Consequently, if confronted by a badly injured patient where shock is suspected, the first step should be to establish a Haemaccel intravenous infusion and run in the first unit of 500 ml as quickly as possible. Some authorities suggest the use of a unit of normal saline as the first i.v. solution, to be followed by Haemaccel. Then a second unit is connected up and run in more slowly, adjusting the rate to fit the patient's clinical picture, blood pressure and pulse. If no blood pressure is recordable or it is very low, say systolic 85, then the second unit needs to be run in quickly as well, whereas a blood pressure of 90 or more indicates that the infusion rate can be slowed down. It is possible to give up to 4 units of Haemaccel en route to hospital to try to maintain the circulating volume, but remember that Haemaccel is not blood, and has no oxygen-carrying capacity. Baskett and Zorab (1977) recommend that the first litre of i.v. fluid in a seriously injured patient should be run through in 20–30 min, although in some cases even faster rates may be needed.

In dealing with an elderly person, however, intravenous fluids should be given more slowly and with caution. The reason for this cautious approach is, ironically, the risk of overloading the circulation. An elderly person's heart is likely to be less effective than a younger person's with the result that heart failure may develop if a litre or more of fluid is given very quickly intravenously.

There is also a need to set up an intravenous infusion when replacement of lost blood is not the immediate aim. For such situations Hartmann's solution or normal saline are recommended as being generally the most useful. For example, acutely ill patients may be very dehydrated (as shown by dry skin which has lost its normal elasticity), and the only way of giving them fluids may well be the i.v. route. Or you may feel that you want an i.v. line as insurance—for instance, if the patient's condition at present is not too bad, but you are worried about future deterioration. In this situation set up the intravenous infusion and run Hartmann's solution slowly.

If the patient has diabetes and is unconscious then an i.v. line is essential because if he or she is hyperglycaemic (too much sugar in the blood) then urgent i.v. rehydration with normal saline will be required, i.e. a 0.9% sodium chloride solution. This is because, in addition to fluid loss, the patient will also have lost large amounts of sodium chloride and other electrolytes (Macleod, 1984). One further fluid the paramedic should have available is 5% dextrose which, like normal saline usually comes in 1 litre bags, dextrose 5% is good for rehydrating a dehydrated patient, but does not contain any electrolytes.

Points to Remember

Provided that the paramedic can gain access to a vein, and has at least 3 units of Haemaccel, plus units of Hartmann's, normal saline and 5% dextrose available, most contingencies should be able to be met. The technique of i.v. cannulation is not easy and needs constant practice. Great attention should be paid to avoiding contamination at all times during the setting up of an intravenous infusion as infection introduced via the venous route can have very serious effects. Paramedics should also remember their own protection, as diseases such as hepatitis and AIDS are bloodborne (see p. 133).

A practical point to remember is to check the expiry date of fluids at frequent intervals as the shelf-life is not infinite. Note, for instance, that Haemaccel carries a date of manufacture rather than an expiry date; according to its manufacturers it has a shelf-life of eight years at room temperature.

Further discussion about i.v. fluids and drugs will be found at appropriate points later in the text.

MAST TREATMENT

This approach to the treatment of shock has gained in popularity in the United States, though not yet to such a great extent in civilian practice in the United Kingdom. The Vietnam war saw the development of what are known as MAST, military anti-shock trousers. They are described by Budassi and Barber (1984) as the single most useful piece of equipment an emergency department can have for the treatment of the patient with multiple injuries or hypovolaemia.

MAST consists of a pair of waterproof, flame-resistant trousers that can be inflated in three chambers, thereby compressing the legs and lower abdomen. The effect of this is to transfuse between 500 and 1000 ml of blood from the periphery to the central circulation where it is most needed in emergency situations. MAST can be applied in about 60 s, and of course the blood thus shunted to the vital heart–lung–brain centres is ready cross-matched, prewarmed to body temperature, and free from any of the hazards of blood transfusion.

An additional bonus of MAST application is that the lower limbs are splinted and compressed, thereby immobilising any fractures and applying pressure to any bleeding wounds. Budassi and Barber recommend the use of MAST, particularly if the systolic pressure has fallen to 80 or below.

MAST should ideally only be left on for 2 h, and only removed slowly and when the lost circulating volume has been replaced. In view of the great advantages that have been reported from the United States, a more widespread use of MAST in the United Kingdom would be welcomed.

References

Baskett P., Zorab J. (1977) Essentials of emergency management. In Easton K. (ed.) *Rescue and Emergency Care*. London: Heinemann.

Budassi S., Barber J. (1984) *Emergency Care*. St Louis: C. V. Mosby Co.

Beverly M., Coombs R. (1985) The management of compound fractures. In Westaby S. (ed.) *Wound Care*. London: Heinemann.

Coco, C. D. (1980) *Intravenous Therapy, A Handbook for Practice*. St Louis: C. V. Mosby Co.

Easton K. (ed.) (1977) *Rescue and Emergency Care*. London: Heinemann.

Fountain W., Westaby S. (1985) The surgical incision and haemostasis. In Westaby S. (ed.) *Wound Care*. London: Heinemann.

Green J. H. (1978) *An Introduction to Human Physiology*, Oxford: Oxford Medical Publications.

Macleod J. (1984) *Davidson's Principles and Practice of Medicine*. Edinburgh: Churchill Livingstone.

Settle J. (1974) *Burns, The First 48 Hours*. St Albans: Smith and Nephew.

Walsh M. (1985) *Accident and Emergency Nursing, A New Approach*. London: Heinemann.

3. Management of Major Trauma

On arriving at the scene of an accident, paramedics should always start their assessment and care by repeating to themselves the letters ABC. This is to remind them of the priorities facing the patient, and to help organise what may be a chaotic situation. Is the airway clear? Is the patient breathing? Can a pulse be felt? We can now look in more detail at some of the other problems the patient may be facing in the aftermath of major injury.

HEAD INJURY

Injury to the head may result in damage to the brain, damage which is usually invisible but potentially far more serious than the obvious injuries, such as scalp lacerations, that one can see. The brain is an immensely complicated and delicate organ sitting in a box of bone, the skull. It is surrounded by three layers or meninges which, working inwards from the skull, are known as the dura mater, arachnoid mater and pia mater. Below the arachnoid mater, in the subarachnoid space, circulates a liquid known as the cerebrospinal fluid (CSF), which also permeates through the brain and surrounds the spinal cord. It acts as a support for these vital structures, maintaining a constant pressure around them. So the skull can be thought of as a watertight box containing brain, blood and CSF (Green, 1978). The significance of this is that any increase in blood volume within the skull will lead to a compression of nerve tissue and a rise in intracranial pressure.

Such changes can have very serious effects on the patient's condition leading to possible permanent damage or even death. It is vital therefore that the paramedic can assess the patient's neurological condition quickly and recognise the signs of rising intracranial pressure. Such a situation is a real emergency and the patient must be taken to the nearest medical facility as soon as possible.

Brain Injury

The pathology of brain injury is very complex, but we can try to sum it up by saying that a blow to the head will produce either a sudden acceleration force (for example, in a stationary person who is hit over the head by a blunt object) or a deceleration force (for example, a motorcyclist coming off his bike and hitting the road). The result is that major forces are transmitted to the delicate structures underneath. These forces are described by Gillingham (1977) as capable of tearing the blood vessels that lie on the surface of the brain, damaging both the vital structures at the base of the brain and the actual substance of the brain and the blood vessels that lie within. All these are possible injuries, and the effect that accompanies any bleeding within the closed box (the skull) is a rise in intracranial pressure. Gillingham points out that any impairment in the airway will lead to a rise in venous pressure within the brain and further increase bleeding. In addition there is a tendency for tissue with elevated carbon dioxide levels to become oedematous (retain fluid), which in turn contributes to rising intracranial pressure.

The picture that emerges then is the possibility of a torn blood vessel bleeding below the skull, either on the surface of the brain or within. The rise in intracranial pressure that accompanies the accumulation of blood from the bleed (*haematoma*) leads to serious complications that compound the damage the brain substance itself has suffered from the forces involved. Fortunately not all head injuries are this severe, however. Gillingham (1977) describes a series of 1135 head injuries admitted to the Royal Infirmary of Edinburgh of which only 79 were classed as serious, the definition being based on a loss of consciousness totalling more than 24 h. It is easy, therefore, to become complacent about head injuries as the paramedic may attend many who develop no significant pathology.

In an effort to try to reduce any such tendencies we should remember that severe injuries when they do occur carry a very high mortality rate. Budassi and Barber (1984) quote mortality rates of 50% and 70% respectively for epidural and subdural haematomas. The dura is the outer of the three meninges referred to earlier that surround the brain; the locations of the two types of bleeds described here are therefore above and below the dura respectively.

Skull Injury

So far we have concentrated on injury affecting the brain, but both the skull and scalp may also be injured. Part of the significance of the presence of a skull fracture lies in the fact that it is an indication of the amount of force involved in the accident (however, 50% of epidural haematomas show no evidence of skull fracture, so it is very misleading to base an estimate of the brain injury purely on the presence or absence of a skull fracture). However, of much greater importance is whether or not the fracture is open – in other words, if there is communication between the fracture and the outside that can be a route for infection to gain access to the bone and structures below, a very serious complication indeed.

Scalp Injury

The scalp has an extremely rich blood supply which means that lacerations in this region can bleed very heavily, contributing to the development of shock in conjunction with other injuries. The elderly are particularly prone to bad scalp wounds sustained when falling. Because of the natural hardening of the arteries that occurs with age (due to the deposition of calcium and a fatty substance known as atheroma) these are not able to react in the same way that a younger person's would, that is by going into spasm to stem the blood loss from the severed end of the artery. Consequently the elderly may suffer profuse blood loss from a scalp wound sufficient to produce shock, with no other injury involved.

ASSESSMENT OF A PATIENT
WITH HEAD INJURY

The first priority is always the airway, as any partial obstruction of the airway, or a rise in blood carbon dioxide levels, may increase intracranial pressure and make the effects of the injury much worse.

Measuring Consciousness

The first effect of rising intracranial pressure is usually a fall in the patient's level of consciousness. Therefore an initial assessment is a crucial benchmark against which subsequent changes will be measured. Consciousness should be monitored throughout the journey to hospital, and a detailed description of any changes given to the staff receiving the casualty. A well-known problem in dealing with head-injured patients involves the so-called 'lucid interval'. Typically, patients recover consciousness after the initial injury and may be quite lucid. However, due to a damaged blood vessel, a slow bleed may occur which produces a rise in intracranial pressure many hours later, severe brain damage and coma. It is just possible that when you are called to head-injured patients who have recovered consciousness, they may be in a lucid interval. Every effort should therefore be made to persuade them to go to hospital even though they may insist that they feel well at the time.

The problem in measuring consciousness is that it is not like a pulse or temperature that can be measured objectively. Two different people should be able to take the same pulse and get very nearly the same answer. However, describing a head injury patient as semiconscious or drowsy is imprecise as these terms may have very different meanings for different people. In an attempt to get round this problem, the Glasgow coma scale was devised and its use is strongly recommended.

The aim of the Glasgow coma scale is to assess the best response the patient can make in terms of motor, verbal and eye-opening actions (Teasdale and Jennet, 1974). Figure 3.1 illustrates the scale in a chart form that could be used in the field. The descriptions used are self-explanatory, the aim being to mark in the best response that the patient is capable of under each of the three sections.

Frequency of Recordings				DATE
....				TIME
		Spontaneously		
	Eyes open	To speech		Eyes closed by swelling = C
		To pain		
C O M A S C A L E		None		
	Best verbal response	Orientated		
		Confused		Endotracheal tube or tracheostomy = T
		Inappropriate Words		
		Incomprehensible Sounds		
		None		
	Best motor response	Obey command		
		Localise pain		Usually record the best arm response
		Flexion to pain		
		Extension to pain		
		None		

Fig. 3.1 Glasgow coma scale

In assessing motor response, the patient may be unresponsive to verbal commands, therefore a painful stimulus is needed to assess response. Walsh (1985) recommends flexing the patient's finger, applying pressure with your thumb at the base of the patient's finger, and with your finger at the tip of the patient's finger. The result should be to bend the finger inwards (flexion) which will produce a painful stimulus (try it on yourself and see!) Note whether the patient responds by trying to knock your hand away (localised pain), bending the arm to withdraw the hand (flexion), extending the arm towards you possibly with marked muscular spasm (extension), or with no response at all. An extensor response indicates damage to the brain stem and its vital centres, and has a very serious prognosis.

Caution: In assessing patients' orientation, asking questions like 'Do you know it is Friday, 9 pm?' is not the best way of finding out because patients may well answer 'yes' to a question phrased in that way without having the faintest idea! Simply ask what day and time it is, then ask where they think they are. If they can answer these questions they are orientated in time and space, if not they are confused.

The next step is to ask what can be remembered of the incident. This may yield vital information, for instance if they were knocked out, for if they were unconscious, there will be a gap in their memory. A short period of unconsciousness, perhaps 30 s or 1 min is a common finding and related to the effects of the blow interrupting the reticuloactivating system in the brain, which among other factors is responsible for maintaining our state of consciousness. Such an injury is referred to as a *concussion*.

Assessing the Pupils

Having assessed the current level of consciousness, and whether there was any loss of consciousness when the injury occurred, the next step is to assess the patient's pupils. They should be equal in size and contract quickly to any light shone into them. This contraction occurs due to the oculomotor nerve stimulating the appropriate muscles to react. This nerve has branches running across the surface of the brain that supply each eye. If there is a rise in intracranial pressure associated with a bleed and haematoma formation, then there is compression of this nerve, which interferes with the movement of the muscle it supplies. The result therefore is that one pupil may start to look bigger than the other and become sluggish to react. If it dilates completely and is totally unreactive, this is a sign of serious brain compression on that side of the skull, while if both pupils are dilated and unreactive, this is a sign of generalised raised intracranial pressure.

Regular assessment of pupil size and reaction is therefore a further guide to the development of any bleeding and rise in intracranial pressure. If pressure rises sufficiently to produce this picture, it will already have had significant effects on the level of consciousness. Consequently a person with unequal pupils, but who is wide awake and fully orientated, is unlikely to be suffering a bleed inside the skull. Other possible explanations are that the pupils are always unequal, or even that the patient may have an artificial eye.

Bleeding from the Ears

The next step is to look for bleeding from the ears, as this may be an indication of a fractured base of skull, but be sure the blood is from *deep within the ear* not from a cut of the lobe. Leakage of CSF from the nose (rhinorrhoea) or ear (otorrhoea) can also occur with base of skull fractures, so should be checked. Any sign of a clear fluid (CSF) oozing from nose or ear should be carefully noted and the information passed on to the medical staff later.

MANAGEMENT OF THE PATIENT
WITH HEAD INJURY

If ABC assessment reveals that patients are unconscious, an oral airway should be inserted to protect their airway, and a high concentration oxygen mask applied running at 4 litres/min. Reference has already been made to positioning patients to protect their airway further if unconscious (p. 4). Note, however, that in head injury there is also a risk of neck injury, so the safest way to proceed is to assume the unconscious patient has a neck injury until proven otherwise (see p. 56 for guidance about moving the patient and immobilising the neck); follow the jaw thrust method (pp. 3–4; see Fig. 1.3) to position the head in clearing the airway.

Wounds

Once the airway is secure, the patient is being well oxygenated and the neck is immobilised, we can turn our attention to other aspects of head injury such as dealing with wounds. A firm pressure dressing is required, with two large dressing pads and a very firmly applied bandage to hold them in place, to control the heavy bleeding that may occur. When applying head bandages, beware of covering the patient's eyes, as this can cause great anxiety and concern especially if consciousness is regained en route to hospital. To assist keeping the bandage in place, use the ears as anchor points, swinging the bandage alternately above and below the ears. A useful tip is to acquire a few 10–15 cm (4–6 in) lengths of Tubigrip bandage, size F. This will fit over the head like a sweat band and hold a dressing neatly in place with considerable compression, provided that the wound is not on top of the scalp. In this case use a skull bandage.

Leaking of Cerebrospinal Fluid

If there is a suspicion of CSF leaking from the nose or ears, try to prevent patients from blowing their nose. If the CSF is leaking there must be passage through to the meninges, and the sudden increase in pressure in the nasopharynx associated with blowing the nose may well force contamination into these vital coverings of the brain itself. Patients with a fractured base of skull are already at risk from serious infection as a result of this passage between the covering of the brain and the outside world, therefore everything possible must be done to minimise this risk. Encourage patients to spit out into a bowl any such fluid they feel dripping into the back of their mouth if they can. Similarly, if the leak is from the ear, lay them on the affected side to facilitate easy drainage and cover the ear with a gauze pad.

Bleeding into the Mouth

Apart from the risks to the airway in an unconscious patient of aspiration, blood also poses another hazard. It is a gastric irritant and therefore if swallowed will produce vomiting, further endangering the patient's airway. The paramedic's nightmare is the person with a head injury, deteriorating level of consciousness, vomiting copiously in the back of an ambulance in a high-speed transfer to hospital. The care of the unconscious head injured patient may be summarised as keeping the airway clear to prevent further brain damage and inhalation of any vomit, and administering oxygen.

There is a valid argument for intubation if the patient is deeply unconscious, and close observation of any changes in the level of consciousness throughout is essential. This information should be passed on to the accident and emergency staff together with any observations of fits (often associated with a depressed skull fracture).

An unconscious patient with both head injury and shock will probably have another injury to account for the shock. It must be emphasised that if the patient is unconscious the paramedic would be wise to assume that the patient has a neck injury until proven otherwise. Transfer to hospital should be as quick as possible, but without endangering the neck by hasty handling. Note use intravenous infusion if BP falling.

FACIAL INJURIES

It is likely that facial injury will accompany head injury, posing significant hazards to the patient's airway. Copious bleeding into the nasopharynx is possible, with the risks of vomiting if swallowed, or asphyxiation if breathed in.

Full Frontal Injuries

While a blow to the side of the face may produce a fracture of the cheek, the full frontal, high energy blow is the most serious, and can produce any one of three characteristic fracture patterns known as Le Fort fractures (types I, II or III) after the French pathologist who first described them (Fig. 3.2). Both Le Fort II and III fractures pose serious risks to the airway. In a type II fracture there is very heavy bleeding into the nasopharynx, and in a type III fracture the front of the face is effectively separated from the rest of the skull, with the result that the airway is greatly at risk due to the now abnormal anatomy. These sorts of injuries are classically associated with front seat occupants in car crashes striking either dashboard or steering wheel with their face in a head-on collision. Seat belt legislation has now greatly reduced the number of such injuries.

Nose Bleeds

Even without such high energy trauma, profuse bleeding from the nose may occur in facial injury. Nose bleeds (epistaxis) can of course occur without any trauma at all, especially in the elderly, and their effect can be very serious in terms both of blood loss and the distress caused. It is not an exaggeration to say that a severe nose bleed may be a life-threatening emergency in an elderly person due to the development of shock. The patient should be treated as for hypovolaemic shock, and the nose bleed treated in line with the recommendations on p. 53.

Trauma to the Eyes

Serious facial trauma may also include the eyes, ranging in severity from lacerations around the eye or a foreign body in it, through to complete loss of the eye itself. Soft tissue swelling may quickly close the eye completely, causing two problems: it will be impossible to monitor pupil size and reaction; and patients may fear they have lost the sight of the eye, or both of them in a bilateral injury, leading to great psychological distress.

Trauma to the Mouth and Teeth

In dealing with mouth injuries, loose teeth or any teeth that have been knocked out are a cause for concern. If inhaled, they

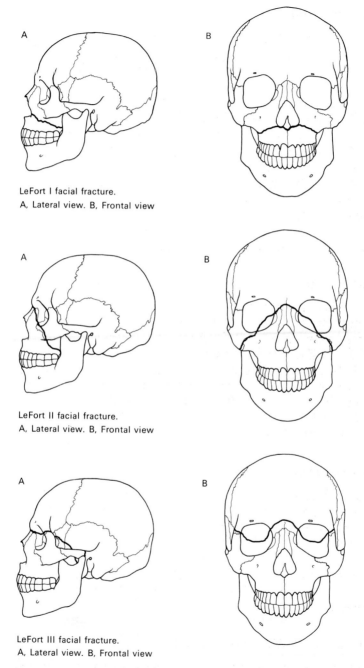

LeFort I facial fracture.
A, Lateral view. B, Frontal view

LeFort II facial fracture.
A, Lateral view. B, Frontal view

LeFort III facial fracture.
A, Lateral view. B, Frontal view

Fig. 3.2   Patterns of fracture, Le Fort types I–III

can lead to serious complications by setting up a focus of infection within the lung, and by blocking one of the bronchioles a tooth may cause collapse of a part of the lung. In extreme cases the airway may be severely impaired if a section of denture is broken off and inhaled.

Management of Facial Injury

Having considered some of the effects of serious trauma on the face, it now remains to see how the paramedic should deal with the situation. As always, the airway is the prime concern. Assess its patency and the patient's respiratory status, also assess the level of consciousness, for any serious blow to the face will have affected the brain. Consider the risk of neck injury (discussed below, p. 54).

Do not be misled by the presence of a lot of superficial blood; the face and scalp have a very rich blood supply. Of more significance than superficial lacerations is the risk of fractures to the facial bones and base of skull. Look for evidence of bleeding from the ears or CSF leakage. Can the patient talk normally? Speech may be impaired by fractures or a dislocation of the jaw, a vital clue. Spend a second assessing the shape of the face, as this can be significantly asymmetrical or flattened with serious facial fractures. Bleeding within the mouth and nasopharynx should also be assessed as this is of great importance in preserving the airway. When looking into the mouth check for any broken teeth or denture, and try to find out where the broken pieces went.

Patient care should be directed to preserving the airway at all times using the techniques discussed earlier. *Caution*: very close attention should be paid to the casualty in transit, and beware complacency as only *one* inhaled blood clot can have catastrophic effects.

Eyes

Check patients' eyesight: is vision normal or can they see double? Double vision may indicate a fracture in the floor of the orbit, the socket in the skull housing the eye. In such a case the muscles that move the eyeball have become trapped in the fracture and cannot coordinate the movement of one eye with the other, hence seeing double. Double vision may also be due to the jarring of the optic nerve by the forces involved in the accident.

If there is trauma to the eyes, the safest way forward is to cover the injured eye with a large gauze swab well moistened with sterile normal saline solution; being wet makes it easier to remove subsequently, and also improves tissue viability. Hold the swab in place with a bandage, though not too tightly. Shaped eye pads are available and are particularly suitable for injuries such as a foreign body which has found its way into the eye. Foreign bodies can lead to loss of vision, especially if they penetrate within the body of the eye. However, a considerable amount of energy is usually required for penetration to occur— for example, glass from a car windscreen, flying debris from industrial processes such as drilling, or fragments propelled by blast after an explosion. The most common form of retained foreign body within the eye is metallic; iron and steel account for between 85% and 98% of intraocular foreign bodies in both civilian and wartime casualties.

The risk of a foreign body should always occur to the paramedic in dealing with facial trauma, and the casual comment, 'I've got something in my eye' should not be passed over lightly. Although there may be no great wound present, there could still be a major threat to the vision of that eye. Much psychological support will be needed in dealing with patients who have suffered trauma around the eyes, as they are likely to be very anxious about their vision and the risk of blindness. Support will also be needed for other patients with facial trauma due to the fear of permanent disfigurement.

Bleeding from the Nose or within the Mouth

This is best dealt with by allowing patients, if possible, to sit upright and telling them to spit out any blood into a receptacle of some sort.

There are two reasons for proceeding in this way (a) to prevent patients swallowing blood which is a gastric irritant and will therefore lead to vomiting; and (b) to measure the amount of bleeding taking place. If the case is a simple nose bleed without any trauma, the best way of controlling the bleeding is to instruct patients to squeeze tightly and continuously for at least 20 min, between finger and thumb, the soft lower part of the nose, below the hard bony middle part. This is a very vascular area, and the usual culprit is a small blood vessel which will often respond well to direct pressure. Ancient 'cures' such as keys down the back of the neck have no place in the modern paramedic's repertoire; the best method is simply direct pressure to the soft part of the nose and instructions to spit out any blood felt trickling down into the back of the mouth.

Severe Trauma to the Face

Severe trauma to the facial region can lead to fractures that extend into the base of the skull. Bleeding may be so severe as to lead to profound shock and great difficulty in maintaining an airway, so much so that intubation may be needed to secure the airway and an intravenous infusion line required to compensate for the bleeding. To repeat, in cases of facial trauma, *never forget the airway*.

NECK AND SPINAL INJURY

Reference has already been made to the problem of unconscious patients suffering from an obvious head injury who may also have a spinal injury that is not apparent. As they are unconscious they will not be able to tell you about any pain in their neck or loss of function in their limbs, but the paramedic should realise that a severe blow to the head may well also affect the neck and spine. You should, therefore, assume a spinal injury until you know otherwise, but at all times never lose sight of the ABC priorities of resuscitation.

The Spinal Cord

The spinal cord is the main nerve trunk system of the body, relaying countless signals from the sense organs and nerve endings up to the brain, simultaneously passing down all the nerve impulses necessary to control movement and a host of other automatic functions such as breathing. This mass of communication so essential for normal functioning all passes through the spinal cord, which in its turn threads its way down through the spinal vertebrae, whose protection it needs as it is very soft. So long as the vertebrae remain neatly aligned, held together by the spinal ligaments, and protecting the spinal cord, all is well. However, if there is fracture of a vertebra, there are two risks: (a) bony fragments being driven into the soft cord causing nerve damage; and (b) the ligaments may become disrupted allowing the vertebrae to slip one on top of the other. This partial dislocation is called a subluxation, and poses a serious threat to the continuity of the spinal cord.

Subluxation may occur without a fracture being present, while the swelling that naturally surrounds any injury may make matters worse by compressing the spinal cord. The ultimate disaster is a complete transection of the cord, although a partial transection is possible, with some nerves escaping damage. The level at which the injury occurs also controls the signs and symptoms that appear. If the injury is above the fifth cervical vertebra (counting down from the head) the outlook is very grave in the case of a complete transection, as this brings total paralysis that includes the diaphragm, essential for breathing.

Assessing the Injuries

In assessing the patient, the paramedic needs to think about the nature of the accident and how likely is neck or spinal trauma as a result. How much energy was involved? How far did the person fall? How fast was the car moving? How far was the pedestrian thrown by the car that hit her? A person thrown 9 m (10 yards) after impact with a moving vehicle who lands head first, as revealed by grazing on the forehead and frontal part of the cranium, is clearly at significant risk of a serious neck injury. What were the direction of the forces? A rotational force often makes serious injury more likely when combined with flexion of the neck. Look for signs of trauma on the face and scalp such as abrasions, which may give a vital clue as to the way the patient hit the ground after falling or being thrown from a car. Consider the possibility of both extension *and* flexion, the so-called whiplash injury associated with being in a car that is hit from behind. Bruising or abrasions on the back may suggest an injury lower down the spinal column.

The great fear in dealing with spinally injured patients is of making a bad situation even worse by careless handling. The spine may be unstable due to ligament damage, yet without serious cord injury. Careless handling at this stage could cause displacement of the vertebrae leading to avoidable damage of the spinal cord, even complete transection.

It is for this reason that the basic principle of treating suspected spinal injury patients is to move them as little as possible, and then only as one unit with no movement of any part of the spine relative to another (see Appendix B, Figs. B.4 and B.5). Only an imminent life-threatening event such as fire or explosion should be allowed to cause the hasty movement of a patient with suspected spine injury. Paramedics must exert their authority and take charge of the situation, as well-meaning but inexperienced attempts at lifting or moving the patient can have the most tragic consequences. *The patient's whole future depends on being correctly handled at this most crucial stage.*

If patients are conscious, check where they feel pain or if they have any unusual tingling sensations (such as pins and needles). Check how much feeling they have in their limbs—diminished, altered, absent or changing sensations are all danger signs. Movement of limbs should also be checked, but only very carefully, remembering that the patient is not going to move a fractured limb. In cases of complete transection of the cord, there will be total paralysis below the level of the injury with loss of sensation. Check the patient's breathing at all times in case the muscles involved in respiration are affected by the cord injury.

Splinting

Before movement is attempted, every effort should be made to splint the suspected injury. A rigid collar should be applied carefully to the neck if this is possible, particularly in the case of persons trapped in the wreckage of a car or under rubble in a collapsed building. The greatest of care should be used in extracting a person from this type of situation (see p. 207) It is recommended that one person is in charge of the lift, and that person should be holding the patient at the site of the suspected injury. At least four or five people are required, one to support the head, one the neck, and ideally three for the trunk. If a scoop (orthopaedic) type of stretcher (see Appendix B, Fig. B.16) is available this should be gently slid under the patient once he or she is lying on flat ground.

Reassurance

The psychological care of patients should not be forgotten as they will understandably be very frightened and all too aware of the possibility of permanent paralysis. Great support is required, but honesty is best, so beware sweeping statements such as 'Of course you will be OK, you will soon get the feeling and use back in your legs.' Rather, a cautious but realistic 'It's early days yet, nobody can tell how much recovery there will be and how long things will take.' It is better to be honest from the start rather than build up false hopes that, when dashed by reality leave victims unable to believe anything they are told again.

Transfer to Hospital

Just as moving the patient *to* the ambulance should be done very slowly and with great care, so should the actual ambulance transfer to hospital. Unless there is any life-threatening emergency, the journey should be made slowly—this is no time for flashing blue lights and sirens, one bad jolt could leave your patient paralysed in all four limbs for life. Drive as if you are driving on eggshells, and when you arrive at the hospital make sure the staff there are fully in the picture before anybody lays a hand on the patient.

The handling of the patient in accident and emergency and transfer to a hospital trolley must be carried out with the greatest care. Ensure that the patient is handed over to a senior nurse who is fully aware of the patient's potential condition and who can supervise management safely. The use of a Hines splint for neck immobilisation is recommended as soft collars offer relatively little support. An alternative is the use of a suction vac-splint which can immobilise the head and neck effectively. Swann, Grundy and Russell (Evans, 1986) recommend the use of a helicopter where difficult or lengthy journeys are involved as this reduces both morbidity and mortality. They also stress the importance of not leaving the patient unattended at any time and of maintaining the head and neck in a stable, neutral position.

CHEST INJURIES

Injuries to the chest can broadly be split into two types: penetrating and non-penetrating. Examples of the former are gunshot wounds or stabbings (Fig. 3.3); examples of the latter include blunt trauma and crush injury. Within the chest is the vital heart–lung system with its associated major arterial and venous network; so injury to this part of the body can therefore have very serious and possibly fatal consequences.

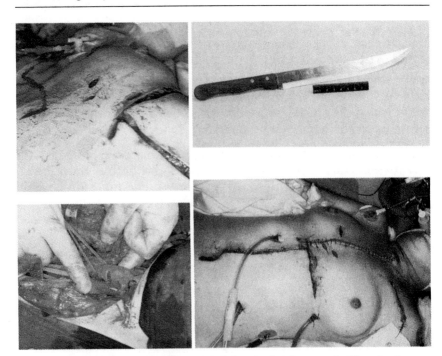

Fig. 3.3   (a) Multiple chest and abdominal stab wounds. The chest
wound lacerated the liver and spleen. (b) Weapon used to assault
patient. (c) Stab wound of the neck which transected the oesophagus
and penetrated the superior vena cava and right lung. (d) The patient
after repair of cardiac, pulmonary, tracheal, oesophageal and hepatic
wounds. The spleen was removed and chest and abdominal drains
inserted

Non-penetrating Injuries

Rib Cage

A logical way of looking at chest injury is to start at the outside
and work inwards. The first major structure encountered is the
rib cage, and blunt trauma here can cause fractures of the ribs. A
fractured rib is extremely painful and will make the patient take
very shallow respirations due to the pain. In itself, however, a
fractured rib is not a life-threatening injury, but if the underlying structures of the lung are involved it becomes a much more
serious situation.

Lungs

The lungs are surrounded by a double-walled sac called the
pleura, and fill with air at each breath by the creation of a pres-

sure within the chest which is less than atmospheric pressure. This is done by expansion of the chest wall and lowering of the diaphragm, the effect being to suck air into the lungs which should both be equally inflated.

Problems start to arise if the pleura is torn so that air and/or blood start to fill this sac surrounding the lungs (Fig. 3.4), resulting in compression of the lung underneath, therefore it cannot expand properly and the amount of oxygen taken in by the patient is reduced. This is known as a *pneumothorax* if air is in the pleura, and a *haemothorax* if there is blood. *This is a serious emergency.*

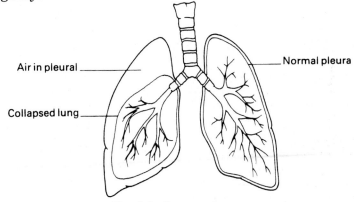

Air in pleural

Normal pleura

Collapsed lung

Fig. 3.4   Pneumothorax

If the tear in the pleura acts as a one-way valve, allowing air to escape into the pleura at each inspiration, but not back at expiration, this is known as a *tension pneumothorax* (Fig. 3.5) and constitutes an immediate life-threatening emergency, the build-up of air in the pleura collapses the lung on the affected side and may then start to affect the other side as well. Further, there will be compression and kinking of vital blood vessels and other structures in the midline of the chest (the mediastinum).

Flail Segment

One further serious complication of blunt chest trauma occurs when several ribs are fractured each in two places forming an isolated section of chest wall known as a flail segment (Fig 3.6). This free section of chest wall will tend to collapse inwards as each inspiration starts to create a pressure within the chest that is less than the atmospheric pressure outside. Consequently the lung underneath will be compressed at the crucial moment when

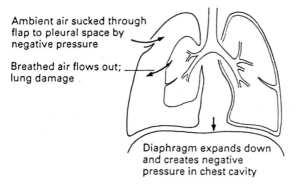

Ambient air sucked through flap to pleural space by negative pressure

Breathed air flows out; lung damage

Diaphragm expands down and creates negative pressure in chest cavity

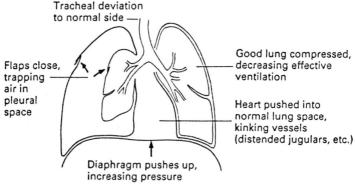

Tracheal deviation to normal side —

Flaps close, trapping air in pleural space

Good lung compressed, decreasing effective ventilation

Heart pushed into normal lung space, kinking vessels (distended jugulars, etc.)

Diaphragm pushes up, increasing pressure

Fig. 3.5   Tension pneumothorax

the patient is in fact trying to expand it, the result being that much less air than normal can enter the lung. Such an injury is often compounded by the presence of a haemothorax.

Assessing Breathing and Colour

In assessing patients who have suffered blunt chest trauma, look at their breathing and colour. Are they showing evidence of cyanosis, is their respiratory effort shallow or laboured? A flail segment will reveal itself by the presence of paradoxical respiration—in other words, a section of chest wall will collapse inwards when the rest of the chest expands, and vice versa. Look for bruising on the chest wall as evidence of injury; tattoo marks from clothing are associated with high energy injury, such as the mark left by a seat belt. Such a situation is often associated with a fractured sternum which will cause the patient considerable central chest pain. If a seat belt had not been worn the injury would have been far more serious. Consider the history of the

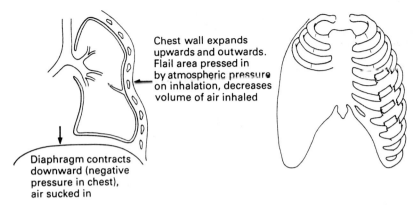

Chest wall expands upwards and outwards. Flail area pressed in by atmospheric pressure on inhalation, decreases volume of air inhaled

Diaphragm contracts downward (negative pressure in chest), air sucked in

Fig. 3.6   Flail chest

accident, was there enough energy involved to cause possible serious internal chest injury? If there is a collapsed section of lung due to a haemothorax or pneumothorax it will reveal itself by being silent when listened to with a stethoscope, but the paramedic must know what normal breath sounds are like first to be able to recognise lung collapse in this way.

Pain and Wounds

If the patient has had significant chest trauma, there may be bruising on the chest wall, but often little else of note. Pain on breathing and respiratory distress, together with the history of the accident, should help in arriving at the conclusion that the patient may have serious internal chest injury. There are also several serious medical conditions that can produce a similar picture (see p. 117).

Positioning is very important in the immediate care of a serious chest injury. Sitting the patient in a partially upright position, turned to the injured side, will give maximum ventilation of the uppermost, uninjured side.

An open, sucking wound must be covered immediately with an airtight occlusive dressing. In certain cases this may actually cause a pneumothorax to develop. If this happens remove the dressing until breathing returns to normal. Re-cover the wound lightly to prevent infection, monitor the breathing, and release the dressing again as necessary. If there is a flail segment the rigidity of the chest wall should be restored by padding, strapping, or by making the patient actually lie on the segment; this latter step may be very painful though. In the absence of an open wound or obvious flail segment, the most likely cause of a severely cyanosed patient will be a tension pneumothorax which may need relieving within minutes if the patient is not to suffer respiratory arrest. This is best accomplished by inserting a large-bore i.v. cannula into the second intercostal space, in the midclavicular line just above the third rib. A hissing sound will confirm entry into the pleural cavity. Whatever the problem, the patient should be given high-concentration oxygen throughout.

Intravenous Infusions

A wise precaution in a patient who has sustained a serious chest injury is to set up an intravenous infusion. The patient may have lost several litres of blood from internal injuries, so the paramedic should always observe for signs of shock developing. The problem then arises of what is the best position for managing the patient: flat with feet up for shock, or sat up to assist breathing? The best solution is probably a compromise in which the legs are elevated to assist venous return, but at the same time the trunk is partly upright, at least 45 °.

The basic principles of management of non-penetrating injury therefore consist of oxygen and correct positioning. Watch carefully both for signs of increasing respiratory distress and the development of shock. An intravenous infusion is a wise precaution early on in case of deterioration later.

Penetrating Injury

Penetrating injury is a potentially serious situation. In addition to the possibility of lung collapse, pneumothorax and/or haemothorax, there is also the risk that the penetrating object may injure a major blood vessel or a vital structure such as the heart or diaphragm, resulting in torrential and rapidly fatal bleed within the chest.

In addition, therefore, to the respiratory support needed as described above, the siting of an intravenous infusion is mandatory, together with vigorous treatment for shock. In addition a sterile occlusive dressing should be applied to the wound site and firmly secured with adhesive tape. The key factor is the depth of penetration rather than the size of the wound. If a stabbing is involved, try to find out the type of weapon, how deep it went, and the angle of entry—vital information that may be available to you at the scene, but not available to the surgeons later (see Fig. 3.3). In view of the potential seriousness of such injuries, it goes without saying that once an intravenous infusion has been established and respiratory support offered—the situation is stable—then a rapid smooth transfer to hospital is essential.

Deceleration Injury

Deceleration injury is found in, for example, a restrained front seat car passenger involved in a high speed collision (Fig. 3.7). The deceleration forces involved are so great that a major blood vessel such as the aorta may suffer a tear in its wall. The patient may be very shocked and moribund with little or no obvious signs of injury. Given the history of a severe deceleration accident, this type of injury should be suspected. Treatment involves giving oxygen and the siting of an intravenous infusion in the usual way. However, beware of bringing the blood pressure up too quickly; if it can be held at a systolic pressure of 90, so much the better. The reason for this caution is that if the blood pressure rises too quickly due to vigorous resuscitation, a damaged section of the aorta can suddenly be forced open and give rise to a massive bleed that will rapidly prove fatal (as aortic aneurysm).

Blast Injury and the Lung

The high pressure blast wave that expands away from an explosion may pass through the chest without producing any marks whatsoever in the skin. However, it may cause catastrophic damage within due to elastic recoil of lung tissue and what is known as the Spalding effect. The alveoli of the lung (the tiny air sacs that form the majority of lung tissue, and where the vital process of gas exchange takes place) are effectively imploded. The damage may be massive and lead to the rapid development of pulmonary oedema—waterlogging of the lungs by tissue fluid. In such a damaged and waterlogged state, the normal exchange of gases cannot take place, and untreated the patient quickly dies.

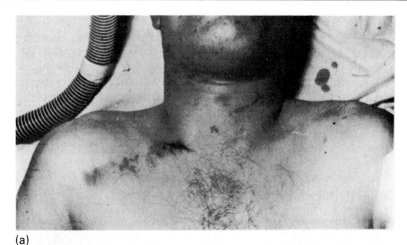

(a)

(b)

Fig. 3.7   Deceleration injuries. (a) and (b) Although the external signs of injury to the patient's neck are not great, the deformation of the steering wheel which struck it shows the force of impact and indicates that underlying tissue damage may be severe. (c), (d) and (e) In this accident the impact was such that the steering wheel was bent against the lumbar spine dividing the jejunum and leaving the pattern of the patient's clothing imprinted on his abdominal wall. (Reproduced by kind permission of Dr H. Proctor, FRCS(Edin).)

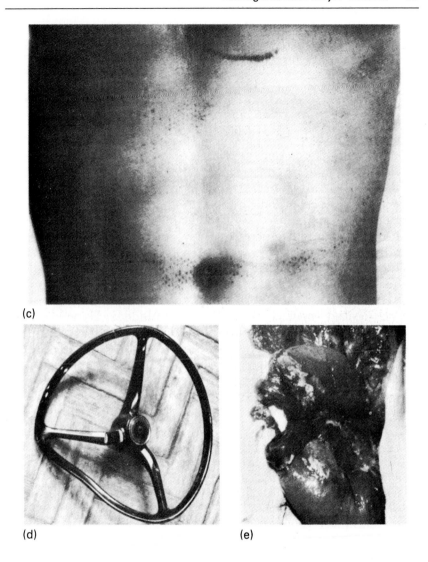

(c)

(d)   (e)

Persons in close proximity to an explosion with no apparent other injury may quickly develop respiratory distress as a result. Evacuation to a medical facility is therefore a high priority, together with close observation in order that any developing respiratory distress may be quickly spotted. The patient must be kept in an upright position, vital to help breathing, and oxygen given from a high concentration mask. *Caution*: beware complacency in dealing with blast casualties who have no apparent injury, for they may have suffered considerable lung damage as a result of the blast wave effect.

ABDOMINAL INJURIES

As with chest trauma, injury to the abdomen may be classified as penetrating or non-penetrating. The penetrating injury seen is commonly either a stab or gunshot wound (see Fig. 3.3) though accidental impalement is sometimes seen, while non-penetrating trauma is usually a severe blow such as might be sustained in a road traffic accident or falling from a height.

The main problems that the patient faces as a result of trauma to the abdomen are (a) either a major internal bleed; or (b) a perforation together with spillage of the contents of one of the organs located there, such as bowel or bladder. Hypovolaemic shock is therefore a major potential problem together with infection from either spillage of bowel contents or the introduction of infection from the outside via a wound. Various other vital functions performed by the organs of the abdominal cavity may be compromised by the effects of trauma.

Signs

In dealing with blunt trauma, look for bruising as a sign of the degree of force involved, and also as a clue as to which organs may be affected. The liver, for example, is a very vascular organ, and bruising here together with a history of a high energy accident should be treated with great suspicion. Bleeding from a damaged liver can quickly lead to a collapsed, moribund patient in a very poor condition. Figure 3.8 shows the location of the main organs in the abdomen and should be a useful guide.

Pain is a crucial symptom that should always be taken seriously. Check if it is localised to one area. Tenderness on palpation is another sign that all is not well, particularly if there is one area that is painful when pressed gently. A very serious sign is generalised abdominal rigidity and severe pain making the patient unwilling to bend in the middle, which indicates that there is widespread inflammation of the peritoneum (the sac

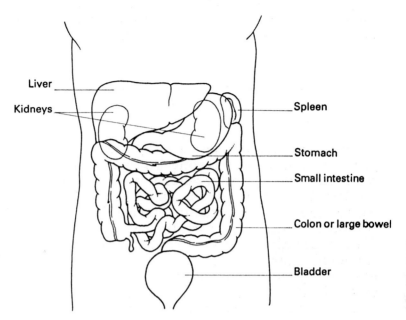

Fig. 3.8   Location of main abdominal organs

that contains the abdominal organs) due to leakage of blood or the contents from a perforated organ.

A close check should be kept on the vital signs of pulse, respiratory rate and blood pressure in order that any development of shock should be spotted as soon as possible.

Initial Management

The first priority in treating the patient should be to resuscitate if there is shock. If there is evidence of high energy trauma, or if transfer to a medical facility is likely to be delayed for any reason, then even though there may not be evidence of shock immediately, it would be wise to set up an intravenous infusion, and run, say, a unit of normal saline slowly as an insurance. In the event of a wound with protrusion of abdominal contents, cover with a large, saline-soaked, sterile gauze dressing. Remember that it is easier to take down a drip than to set one up on a collapsed patient.

The patient should be kept nil by mouth, neither solid food nor liquids should be allowed as they would complicate the anaesthetic if emergency surgery is required. Vomiting is a potential problem so make sure that a vomit bowl is available during transfer. Do not hesitate to give the patient Entonox (see Appendix B, Fig. B.6) if there is pain. Try to obtain a good history if possible for the medical staff receiving the patient.

If the patient has sustained a penetrating injury, then most of the comments made under the section on penetrating injury to the chest will apply (see pp. 62–63). Do not be fooled by a small wound, it is the *depth* of penetration that matters together with the parts of the patient's anatomy that were encountered en route by the offending article. There is obviously a much greater risk of shock developing, with the added complication of the introduction of infection from the outside. The patient should also be kept nil by mouth at all costs, as it is highly probable that a general anaesthetic will be required as in all but the most minor of stabbing cases the surgeon will wish to explore the wound track.

In transferring cases of abdominal injury, allow patients to adopt the position that they find most comfortable, and at all times be vigilant for the development of shock. A well-looking casualty can deteriorate very quickly into a critical condition as a result of internal injury.

TRAUMA AND HIGH VELOCITY PROJECTILES

A high velocity projectile is usually taken to mean an object travelling faster than the speed of sound (1200 km/h; 1100 ft/s), be it a bullet or piece of shrapnel or any other debris from an explosion. The significance of this speed is concerned with the effects that the object has on travelling through the air. It will build up in front of it a pressure wave that can exert extremely high pressures for a fraction of a second, while behind the object there is something akin to a vacuum, resulting in a dramatic drop in pressure fractionally later that will suck contamination into the wound after the object has passed through. The dramatic pressure changes that occur as a high velocity projectile passes through body tissue produce a cavity 30 to 40 times the diameter of the projectile (Owen-Smith, 1985), and causes immense damage; the denser the tissue the worse the damage will be, thus organs such as the liver and brain and tissues like muscle and bone are very sensitive to damage. Complicating the picture further is major contamination caused by the suction effect of negative pressures in the wake of the projectile.

In practical terms, the bullet from a handgun can be considered a low velocity projectile that will not produce such effects, typical velocities being of the order of 770–1100 km/h (700–1000 ft/s), even if the weapon is an automatic. However, a typical rifle fires a lighter projectile at much greater velocities, a military rifle having a muzzle velocity of 2850 km/h (2600 ft/s; bullet weight about 10 g). The Colt Armalite fires a much lighter bullet (3.5 g) at 3560 km/h (3250 ft/s), similar to the modern Russian AK74 (currently in use in Afghanistan). It is the very high velocity of such bullets that makes the weapons so fearsomely effective, being capable of producing severe wounding at ranges of around 1 km (over half a mile) compared to the much shorter ranges (less than 90 m; 100 yards) at which pistols can cause serious wounding. In addition to rifle bullets, the shrapnel from an explosion also has a high velocity; however, due to the lack of streamlining, such fragments will quickly become low velocity projectiles at a distance from the point of explosion. In combat, Owen-Smith (1985) describes some 80% of casualties as being caused by fragments from explosive devices. Modern terrorists are well aware of this effect, as is shown by IRA bombs packed with nails, ballbearings and other objects, creating a great number of serious injuries on detonation.

The effect of bomb blast waves on the lungs has already been described (p. 63). It should be noted that even someone sheltering behind a solid object is still vulnerable to the sudden pressure changes associated with the blast wave. A common finding amongst bomb blast survivors is deafness due to perforated eardrums.

In dealing with casualties, the paramedic needs to find out if possible what sort of weapon was used. A small entry and exit wound the size of your little finger may conceal massive damage to a large volume of tissue within if the bullet was from a high velocity weapon. An intravenous infusion and vigorous resuscitation will be needed together with an occlusive dressing to prevent further contamination of the wound. The patient should be kept strictly nil by mouth as major surgery will be required very quickly. Pain relief is a high priority.

In dealing with shrapnel injuries from explosions it is safer to assume that if the person was close then the culprit was a high velocity projectile. Sometimes the forces involved may be sufficient to cause the traumatic amputation of a whole limb or part of it. Such injuries are common in dealing with the survivors of explosions. Owen-Smith (1985) describes how in explosions in confined spaces about 25% of the dead or seriously injured will have suffered traumatic limb amputation. Pain relief, vigorous resuscitation with oxygen and intravenous infusion fluids, an occlusive dressing, and psychological support if conscious are urgently required before speedy casualty evacuation.

In UK civilian practice, the gunshot wounds most likely to be encountered are those caused by the use of a shotgun. They tend to be devastating at close range with massive tissue damage and contamination. Wounds can be fatal at considerable range. As with all gunshot wounds, care should be taken to ensure that vital evidence, such as clothing, is not lost in transferring the casualty to hospital. Shotguns are frequently used in suicide, with characteristic patterns of wounding to the head and face, the so-called 'sites of election'.

References

Budassi S., Barber J. (1984) *Emergency Care*. St Louis: C.V. Mosby Co.

Evans C. R. (eds.) (1986) *ABC Resuscitation*. London: BMA.

Gillingham F. J. (1977) Head and spinal injuries. In Easton K. (ed.) *Rescue and Emergency Care*. London: Heinemann.

Green J. H. (1978) *Introduction to Human Physiology*. Oxford: Oxford Medical Publications.

Owen-Smith M. (1985) Wounds caused by the weapons of war. In Westaby S. (ed.) *Wound Care*, London: Heinemann.

Teasdale G., Jennet B. (1974) The Glasgow coma scale. *Lancet*, **2**: 81.

Walsh M. H. (1985) *Accident and Emergency Nursing, A New Approach*, London: Heinemann.

4. Trauma Affect   の
the Limbs

INTRODUCTION

Trauma to the limbs can involve wounds, soft tissue and joint injuries; and fractures. Each of these is dealt with in turn.

WOUNDS AND LACERATIONS

The majority of wounds affect the limbs, especially the peripheries such as fingers. Many classification schemes have been devised to describe wounds but, as Westaby (1985) states, they do not deserve the importance that has been attached to them. He considers two factors only of importance: Is the wound sterile or contaminated? Has there been loss of tissue? The basis for this method of looking at wounds is simply that these are the two cardinal factors that will govern any subsequent treatment.

Infection

In practice, most of the wounds that will be encountered by the paramedic are contaminated with bacteria and therefore prone to the risk of infection. It is only a matter of degree how much infection is present. What is of great significance is the presence of *anaerobic* bacteria, meaning they can live without free oxygen. Two common anaerobic strains of bacteria give rise to the much-feared conditions of gas gangrene (*Clostridium perfringens*) (Fig. 4.1) and tetanus which still carry a high mortality cause they are anaerobic these bacteria will thrive in ds that are closed over. Consequently in grossly contami- ted wounds, the tendency is to leave them open for several days, then close them by delayed primary suture perhaps 3 or so

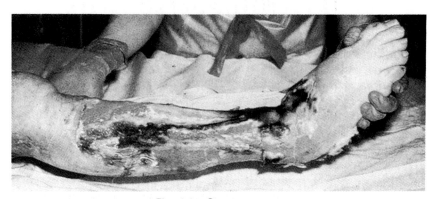

Fig. 4.1   Gas gangrene

days later when surgeons are satisfied that surgical excision and cleansing of the wound has removed all such organisms. If there is relatively little risk of infection then the wound can be thoroughly cleaned out and closed straightaway.

Tissue Loss

In dealing with tissue loss, the second factor in considering wounds, it will be obvious that a clean-cut wound or laceration will usually entail no loss of tissue, therefore the wound edges may be approximated and the wound closed by either suture or the increasingly popular adhesive strip method (such as Steri-strip).

Tissue loss can range from minor abrasions through to degloving injuries where, for example, the tissue covering a whole foot may be stripped off by shearing forces. Medical treatment will vary from the conservative approach of dressing the wound and relying on the body to regenerate new tissue, to skin grafting in more major cases. Sometimes the damage is irreparable and amputation becomes the only possible treatment (Fig. 4.2). Chapter 5 deals with burn injuries from this perspective.

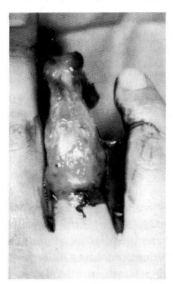

Fig. 4.2   Severe tissue loss caused by an avulsion injury to the ring finger. The ring had been caught up in moving machinery

Assessing the Wound

As with all emergency work, the paramedic should begin by assessing the situation. Find out what was the offending article that caused the wound. If it is still buried in the limb, resist the temptation to try to extract it as you will cause the patient unnecessary pain, and possibly further bleeding, and may also do unknown damage. It is best to dress the wound around the protruding object, thereby avoiding the danger of forcing it further into the wound. Removal of objects from wounds is best carried out in hospital under controlled conditions, where the patient can be given pain relief.

In examining the wound, estimate blood loss and the type of bleeding. Blood loss is notoriously difficult to estimate as a little bit goes a long way—think of the last time you dropped a pint milk bottle! Is the bleeding venous or arterial in origin? Venous bleeding tends to be less severe and consists of a steady ooze of dark-coloured blood (venous blood is poor in oxygen, hence the colour). Arterial bleeding is characterised by a bright red colour (rich in oxygen) and, most important, is pulsatile in nature, the blood vessel spurting blood with each heartbeat.

Your assessment should also include a check for any other

structures that may be exposed in the wound or have been severed by the wounding agent. Tendons, the tough elastic fibres that attach muscles to bone, may be visible as yellowy strands in the wound, and if severed will usually need surgical repair for the patient to regain full use of their limb. Sensation and function of the limb beyond the wound site should be checked as damage to nerves and tendons will be revealed by a loss of sensation and movement and necessitate surgical repair; in view of this, keep the patient nil by mouth.

Controlling Bleeding and Applying Dressings

Bleeding is usually easy to deal with, direct pressure on the wound and elevation of the limb will control most bleeds. Keeping the limb still (lie the patient down where necessary!) also reduces bleeding—exercise obviously requires a larger blood supply than rest. As mentioned above, tourniquets are unnecessary, in fact positively dangerous, and will cause serious damage due to the lack of blood supply. If a tourniquet is not properly applied, the effect will be to increase bleeding. While the venous return is stopped the pressure within the arterial system is such that arterial blood still gets through, so the limb becomes engorged with blood and bleeding increases.

A large dressing pad should be applied to the wound to prevent the introduction of further contamination, and to absorb any further oozing. This may be held in place by a firm pressure bandage to control bleeding. Beware applying your pressure bandage overenthusiastically, however, for you may well end up with a tourniquet. After application, check the colour of the skin beyond the wound to make sure it remains normal; if it is very pale the bandage is too tight. Check also for a pulse. In dealing with a grossly contaminated wound, irrigation with sterile normal saline before applying the dressing will have two advantages: (a) flushing away the worst of the contamination; and (b) keeping the tissue moist underneath the dressing, which makes it easier to remove and also improves tissue viability.

This issue of dressing removal raises the question of the use of a non-adherent dressing actually in contact with the wound surface. Your patient will certainly appreciate this as it can be extremely painful to remove a dressing that has become stuck to the wound. Remember though to make sure you have a thick absorbent pad behind the non-adherent dressing (such as Melolin) to soak up any oozing.

Checklist for Handling Wounds

The following is a useful checklist:

(1) Find out how the wound was caused.
(2) Look at it, check depth, area and involvement of other structures (remember that some people may faint at this stage!)
(3) Control bleeding with direct pressure and elevation above the level of the heart.
(4) Apply firm pressure dressing (not too tight!) and elevate the limb.
(5) Reassure the patient and offer psychological support.
(6) Keep the patient nil by mouth in case a general anaesthetic is needed.
(7) Transfer to medical facility.
(8) Enquire when the patient last had an antitetanus injection. Tetanus is a potentially fatal disease which may develop when spores of the *Clostridium tetani* bacteria are introduced into a wound from the outside environment. Prevention is far better than cure as we all know. Patients should therefore always be advised to attend hospital for a course of antitetanus injections or a booster injection even for a trivial scratch, as there are documented cases of tetanus originating from such minor injuries as a rose thorn pricking the skin. If the patient has no antitetanus protection from a previous course, an injection of Humatet may still be given; this is the ready-made human antibody to the tetanus bacteria which provides protection against this very serious disease developing.

See p. 33 for the treatment of hypovolaemic shock if the wound is severe enough to cause shock to develop.

JOINT INJURIES

Joints are essential for limb movement and normally consist of regular bone surfaces covered in smooth cartilage which can glide over each other with the minimum of friction. The joints are lubricated by synovial fluid, just as engine parts are lubricated by oil, and held together by very tough tissue called ligament.

As joints are usually very stable structures, it requires a high energy injury to dislocate a joint totally, i.e. where the ligaments holding the joint together are torn, and the joint surfaces that should be opposed to one another are completely separated. Slightly less force produces a subluxation injury in which the joint surfaces are still partly in contact. Most commonly seen is an injury involving much less energy, the effect of which is to tear some of the individual fibres within the ligaments surrounding the joint. This produces a sprain, characterised by pain, and some swelling due to the accumulation of tissue fluid around the damaged area. Joint dislocation is recognised by the abnormal appearance of the joint, severe pain, and usually a total lack of movement.

In assessing a patient who has suffered a joint injury, obtain the history first. How much force was involved and what was the direction of the force? Check sensation and circulation beyond the joint, is the limb warm (compare with the other limb to check)? What is its colour and can you feel a pulse? It is possible in a dislocation that an artery or nerve may be trapped which would be an indication for urgent removal to hospital and reduction of the dislocation to save the limb. Find out if the patient can move the joint, but do not try to force any movement. Check how much pain there is.

Having decided that there is a significant joint injury, try to support the limb to minimise any stress on the joint and allow the patient to put it in the position he or she finds most comfortable. Offer Entonox (see Appendix B, Fig. B.6) for pain relief, and keep the patient nil by mouth in case an anaesthetic is required.

Dislocation of Fingers or Toes

Resist the temptation to 'just give it a quick pull'. Transfer the patient to hospital with the injured digit elevated to reduce swelling. Dislocation can be reduced under local anaesthetic. The patient will need an x-ray to check if there is any fracture associated with the injury.

Elbow Injury

This may involve fracture through the supracondylar region of the humerus (see p. 85). There is a threat to the brachial artery supplying blood to the lower arm and also to nerves. If there is any doubt about the circulation, get the patient to hospital as quickly as possible. This is a well known injury in young children, usually after falling from a tree or similar height. Support the arm with a sling.

Shoulder Dislocation

This is a common injury. Considerable force is needed to produce it, but it can recur with increasing ease. The smooth rounded contour of the shoulder is lost as the head of the humerus slips forward and down out of its socket (Fig. 4.3a), and is replaced by a characteristic angular appearance (Fig. 4 3b). Support the arm so there is no weight on the shoulder (sling or pillow), offer Entonox as this is a very painful injury. Patients can range from

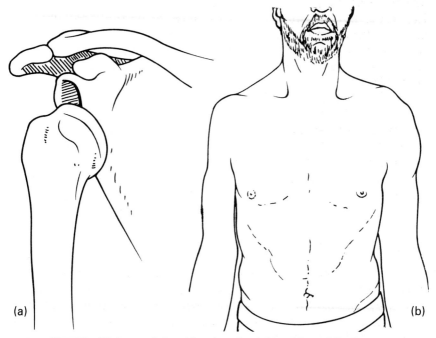

(a)   (b)

Fig. 4.3   Dislocated shoulder showing (a) position of displaced humerus, and (b) the characteristic angular appearance ('flattening')

an 18-year-old rugby prop forward to an 88-year-old grand-mother. If possible lay the patient face down with the arm over the side of the trolley, as this may reduce the dislocation sponta-neously. Reduction is best done as soon as possible since the longer it is left the more difficult it may be.

Sprained Ankle

This is usually caused by stumbling awkwardly. Considerable swelling may occur and the injury can be very painful, so much so that the person is unable to walk on it. The greater the amount of energy involved the more likely it is that there will be a frac-ture as well, for example, in running as opposed to walking. El-evation of the ankle above the level of the heart is required to minimise the swelling, which in its turn will reduce the amount of pain experienced. If the ankle is stable, support it on a pillow, though if there is evidence of instability, severe pain or localised bony tenderness (see p. 81), immobilisation of the ankle in tran-sit with splintage is required. The use of cold compresses may re-lieve some of the swelling and pain, provided that they are not too tightly applied.

Dislocated Ankle

Severe violence is required for such an injury, which is usually accompanied by fractures of the tibia and fibula, sometimes open. Further consideration to this injury is given in the section on fractures, as is a closed injury with subluxation of the joint and associated fractures (p. 86).

Dislocation of the Patella

Dislocation of the patella (kneecap) is often described by the lay person as a dislocation of the knee. However, dislocation of the knee is a rare, high energy injury such as that caused by a high speed road traffic accident (RTA), while dislocation of the patella is a low energy injury associated with congenital joint weakness and other abnormalities in the anatomy of the knee region (Adams, 1976). The injury is common in teenage girls and pres-ents as a locked knee in a position of flexion, with the patella displaced laterally to the side of the knee. Support the leg in the most comfortable position and transfer the patient to hospital where the dislocation can be reduced simply by pushing the patella back where it belongs after appropriate sedation and pain relief. If the patient is given adequate Entonox to relieve pain the ensuing relaxation may be sufficient to achieve a spontaneous reduction of the dislocation en route to hospital.

Dislocation of the Femur

This injury tends to occur in two groups of patients. The younger age group, such as motorbike riders, are usually the victim of high energy accidents. The head of the femur may be driven through the acetabulum, the smooth socket into which it fits, with the joint capsule intact, or it may be driven out of the back of the acetabulum. This latter injury is typical if the victim was sitting at the time of impact, such as a front seat passenger in a car. An older age group of patients may suffer this injury after hip replacement surgery, as the joint capsule is weakened after surgery, and it is possible for the new head of femur to dislocate in some cases.

The affected leg will be shortened and rotated internally. Pain may be severe, especially in the case of a high energy injury, and the patient is unable to move the leg. This clinical picture, together with the type of history described above, should be strongly suggestive of a hip dislocation.

It is important for the leg to be well immobilised before transfer, using either a Fracpac (see Appendix B, Fig. B.3) or splinting with the other leg (see p. 82). Always remember to include padding between the bony prominences of the knees and ankles for protection. The patient should be kept nil by mouth as a general anaesthetic may be needed to reduce the dislocation.

As can be seen from this discussion of some common injuries, the basic principles involved are to check that the circulation and nerve supply beyond the injury are not impaired (if they are, transfer to hospital is of the highest priority), support the limb and immobilise the joint, then give pain relief with Entonox. Reassurance and psychological support are very important in these often painful injuries.

FRACTURES

Just as there are various schemes for categorising wounds, so it is with fractures. However, the paramedic in the field need not be too concerned with academic orthopaedic exercises, and should instead look at fractures from the point of view of: are they open or closed, and how stable is the limb? The former point is of great importance due to risk of infection, while the latter point obviously has implications for handling and moving the patient.

Cause of Fractures

When a bone fractures, there will always be bleeding from the exposed ends of the bone. In the case of large bones this may be sufficient on its own to cause shock without any other injury or wounds. In a closed fracture of the femur 1 litre (2 pints) of blood will be lost, while in fractures of the pelvis blood loss may be up to 2 litres.

This blood will seep into the surrounding tissues causing swelling to occur; the more swelling there is, the more painful the injury will tend to be.

The forces producing the fracture may have acted along the axis of the bone with the result that there is little displacement, the bone ends being crunched together into what is known as an *impacted fracture*. Examples are associated with a fall on the outstretched hand leading to an impacted fracture of the lower radius or the neck of humerus in the elderly. Such an injury is relatively stable in that the bone ends will not move much in relation to each other.

If, however, the force has acted across the bone, the probability is that the fracture line will also run across the bone leading to an injury that is displaced. The danger here is that vital structures such as nerves or blood vessels may be trapped by the displaced bone, and lead to the loss of the limb in severe cases as the distal part is deprived of its blood supply. Great care will be needed in moving the limb as it will be very unstable. Such injuries often show major deformity due to the displacement of the bone ends. If a twisting force is involved, the resulting fracture will be of a spiral nature, a relatively stable injury, with much less obvious deformity.

An open fracture is defined as one where there is communication between the outside and the fracture site. This of course leads to the risk of infection, either of the soft tissues or of the bone itself, osteomyelitis, a very serious complication that is still extremely difficult to treat. It only needs a small puncture wound where a sliver of bone has penetrated the skin from within at the moment of impact, for the injury to be treated as an open fracture.

Assessment of Fracture

First obtain a history: was there enough violence to break a bone? Gently examine the injured limb, remembering that there may be more than one fracture, for example, as a result of a serious fall, there may be an obviously badly displaced fracture of the wrist. However, the other wrist might also be broken, the patient may have a further fracture higher up the arm.

If the fracture is displaced there may be obvious deformity, but a lot of fractures are not displaced. The cardinal sign that should make you suspect a fracture is known as *localised bony tenderness*; if you gently press the fracture site, the patient will experience pain where you are pressing. Thus an undisplaced fracture of the tibia or an impacted fracture of the radius will be revealed when you press gently over the fracture site, even though there may be no obvious deformity.

Check to see if there is a wound near the fracture, as even a small puncture wound is sufficient to make it an open fracture. Then look beyond the injury to the rest of the limb, check sensation and blood supply to eliminate the possibility of nerve or blood vessel damage.

Assess the patients' understanding of the problem and their degree of pain. Some patients may not understand that they have a possible fracture and will therefore not be very cooperative (for example, a young child or somebody who is confused, or someone who does not speak English). How are they reacting to the injury? Chapter 11 gives advice on how to handle the psychological aspects of patient care.

Immobilisation

Always handle suspected fractures very gently. Apart from reducing pain, this also minimises the risk of further damage being caused by the bone ends within the limb. The limb should be fully supported at all times. The next step is to immobilise the fracture so that the patient can be transferred without causing avoidable pain or damage to the limb. If there is a wound this should be dressed immediately to reduce the risk of contamination and infection at the fracture site.

In splinting fractures one or two basic principles should be followed at all times. First, make sure that there is plenty of padding to protect any bony prominences such as the inside of the knees or the ankles. Do not apply too tightly, as there is likely to be considerable swelling around the injury, so always check the circulation beyond the fracture to make sure it is adequate. The application of traction to closed fractures while splinting often provides pain relief in the long term due to the improved alignment of the bone. Finally, explain to the patient what you are doing and why, as this will help gain their cooperation and make life a lot easier for everybody.

A useful tip is to carry with you a large pair of strong scissors. There will be occasions when you cannot see the fracture site, and it is too painful for the patient to get undressed, therefore the only way of seeing the injury is to cut off clothing with the scissors (try, for example, to cut trousers along the seams). Before you do this though, explain why it is necessary and obtain the patient's consent. Usually the patient will not object, as often clothes are torn and ripped anyway as a result of the accident. If, however, the patient flatly refuses to let you cut the clothing, then respect his or her wishes. As a precaution it might be advisable to get your partner to witness this refusal.

Give patients as much Entonox as necessary for pain relief, as fractures are very painful injuries. If patients have sustained a head injury, you may have a dilemma in view of what has been said about observing the level of consciousness, given that Entonox will itself cause drowsiness. If the patient's level of consciousness is impaired, it is safest not to give Entonox (Zorab and Baskett, 1977). In such a situation, they would probably not be able to self-administer it anyway. If, however, they are fully awake and alert, in pain, and oriented in time and space, consideration should be given to allowing patients the use of Entonox, as its effects wear off within a few minutes, so it is still possible to check regularly the level of consciousness.

It should be emphasised that if the circulation or nerve supply to the limb beyond the fracture site is impaired, the removal of the patient to hospital becomes a matter of the greatest urgency, as emergency treatment may be needed to save the limb. In some cases the limb may be lost as a result of this fracture complication.

A more detailed discussion of splinting will be found on p. 256. However, it is worth mentioning here the use of *vacsplints*, strongly recommended by the present author elsewhere for use in accident and emergency departments (Walsh, 1985), as they may also be used in the field provided that a source of suction is available, as it is in most ambulances. A vacsplint is simply a plastic bag full of polystyrene beads with a one-way valve attached. When suction is applied, air is sucked out of the bag which then collapses around the limb and becomes rigid. The splint is moulded to the exact shape of the limb and is only under atmospheric pressure, greatly reducing the risk of tissue injury due to compression. The splint is transparent to x-rays, so it need not be completely removed when the patient reaches the accident and emergency unit, saving considerable pain and discomfort. The stability gained and the ease of application make them well worth serious consideration.

Checklist for Handling Fractures

The basic principles are as follows:

(1) Obtain the history.
(2) Gain access to the injury site, assess the injury, the limb beyond the injury site, and the rest of the patient.
(3) Dress any wounds, and explain what you are doing and why.
(4) Keep the patient nil by mouth in case anaesthetic is required later.
(5) Offer Entonox.
(6) Splint limb.
(7) Transfer to hospital, checking circulation continuously.

Fractures of the Forearm

Falling on an outstretched hand leads to fracture through the

supply. Make sure you can find the pedal pulse to check blood supply to the foot at all times. (see Fig. 4.6). Elevate the injured leg, offer Entonox, give nil by mouth. Injury may be of a twisting nature (common in sports such as football) leading to a spiral fracture which is relatively stable and undisplaced, so there may be little deformity. If the injury involves a gaping wound then an intravenous infusion should be set up and commenced in anticipation of shock developing. Such an injury could easily result in the loss of 1 litre of blood or more; a closed fracture may lead to the loss of approximately ½ litre of blood.

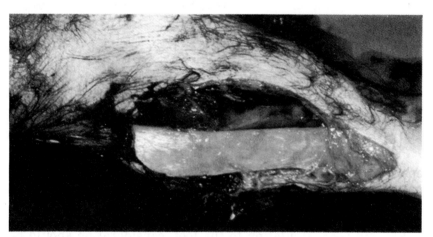

Fig. 4.7   Open fracture of the tibia.

Fractures of the Femur

There are, broadly speaking, two types of femoral fractures; the high energy type that tend to affect younger people; and the very low energy type that affect the elderly, and are more a result of thinning and disease of the bone due to advanced age. In this latter group the fracture is usually high in the femoral neck region rather than the shaft of the bone (Fig. 4.8).

If there is a femoral shaft fracture there will tend to be shortening of the affected limb by as much as a few centimetres, and pronounced swelling of the thigh due to the large blood loss involved. Pain will be severe. The leg will need splinting (see p. 82). If there is likely to be a delay in moving the casualty, an intravenous infusion should be set up as the blood loss is sufficient to cause shock, and an open fracture of the femur may lose twice

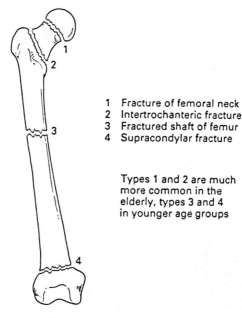

1 Fracture of femoral neck
2 Intertrochanteric fracture
3 Fractured shaft of femur
4 Supracondylar fracture

Types 1 and 2 are much
more common in the
elderly, types 3 and 4
in younger age groups

Fig. 4.8   Fracture of the femur

as much blood as a closed fracture (2 litres as opposed to 1 litre).
Run Haemaccel in slowly and check pulse and blood pressure
every 15 minutes if there is a delay, speeding up the intravenous
infusion rate if needed. Oxygen should be administered during
transfer to hospital as part of the treatment to prevent shock.

A fracture in the region of the femoral neck is a very common
injury in the elderly, the average age of such patients being over
80, and the overwhelming majority being female (Walsh, 1985).
The patient will be found to have a shortened leg on the affected
side which is externally rotated. Bleeding from the femur in this
region is slight, and therefore shock is not a problem. Splint one
leg against the other and handle very gently; old people may be
very frail.

There are many psychological and social problems in dealing
with elderly patients, not just after a fall and a fracture, but in a
variety of other emergency situations, so remember the following points. Explain what you are doing and why, where you are
taking the patients and what will happen to them, this will help
to reduce confusion, a major problem in the elderly. Remember
they may have a hearing aid or glasses, without which their abil-

ity to communicate and understand will be impaired. They may live alone, so who contacts the next of kin (if there are any), locks the house up and looks after the pet goldfish? These are just some of the possible social problems that start to become apparent and must be dealt with. Any social background information that you can give accident and emergency staff will be gratefully received.

Fractures and Children

Children's bones are different from adults as the child is still growing. They are softer and have a region of growth at either end known as the epiphysis. Because they are much softer than adult bones they behave differently when subject to trauma, having a tendency to bend and partly break, like the branch of a tree (hence the name greenstick fracture, usually used to describe fractures in children). Very young children, under the age of 2, have bones so soft that it is very difficult indeed for them to fracture, a fact that is of significance in considering child abuse. Given the inquisitive and adventurous nature of children, they are frequently involved in accidents that lead to fractures (see p. 154 for advice on handling the psychological side of their injury, which is just as important as the physical).

The physical care of a suspected fracture in a child is much the same as that described for adults, always remembering to keep them nil by mouth as a general anaesthetic may well be required to manipulate the fracture into a correct position.

References

Adams C. (1976) *Outline of Fractures.* Edinburgh: Churchill Livingstone.

Walsh M. (1985) *Accident and Emergency Nursing, A New Approach.* London: Heinemann.

Westaby S. (1985) *Wound Care.* London: Heinemann.

Zorab, J. S. M., Baskett, P. J. F. (1977) *Immediate Care.* London: W. B. Saunders.

5. Burns

INTRODUCTION

Burn injury involves destruction of skin and possibly underlying tissue to various depths, depending on the burning agent, amount of heat and length of contact. Commonly seen causes of burns are steam, hot water, and flames; less common causes are chemicals, an electrical current, or radiation (bad sunburn, for example). A pulse of thermal radiation is released whenever there is an explosion, this may cause flash burns to exposed skin, and could also be considered an example of a radiation burn, although the term is usually understood in terms of ionising radiation.

Whatever the cause the effect is the same: energy is released into the surface layers of the body resulting in the destruction of tissue to varying depths. Various classification schemes have been proposed for burns, but little common agreement has been reached about a standard classification. It is best therefore to ignore talk of first and second degree burns as these mean different things to different people.

DEPTH OF BURN

As far as the treatment of burns is concerned, what matters is the depth of the burn and the surface area affected. Taking the depth first, this does offer a meaningful classification of burns which has become widely accepted (Sanders, 1985; Fig. 5.1). If

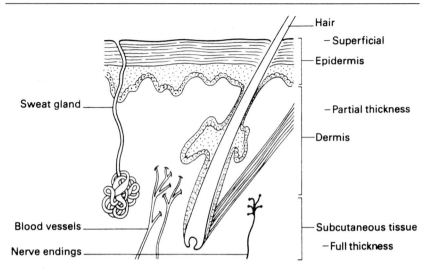

Fig. 5.1   Cross-section of skin to show depth of burn

the burn is of sufficient depth that it has destroyed all the skin, hair follicles and glands (for example, sweat glands) it is known as a *full-thickness burn* and will require skin grafting for healing to occur, without the formation of scar tissue causing serious long-term impairment of function. If, however, only the superficial layers of the skin are involved (such as in sunburn), it is logically known as a *superficial burn* which will heal itself very quickly as the deeper cells that regenerate new skin are intact. Somewhere in between the two is a *partial-thickness burn*, where the sweat glands and hair follicles are preserved, though the outer layers of skin are lost leaving only the deeper dermis. From the islands of surviving tissue around the hair follicles and glands, new skin can grow out over the burnt area in time, provided it is kept free from infection and mechanical injury.

AREA OF BURN

The second factor is the area of burn (see Fig. 5.2). The burnt area will lose fluid from the damaged tissue over a period of 24–48 h. This fluid is very similar to plasma, and if sufficient fluid loss occurs the result will be hypovolaemic shock. The amount of loss depends on the area of the burn. Sanders (1985) pointed out that below 10% of surface area burnt serious problems do not occur. But with a 15% burn in an adult, or a 10% burn in a child, shock is likely to develop. Initial shock may be made worse by pain.

BURN FEATURES

Burns present a major infection risk; this is one of the major battles that have to be fought in the treatment of the patient. They are also extremely painful, except ironically in the case of a full-thickness burn, for here the nerve endings in the deeper tissues will have been destroyed. This in fact represents a diagnostic test for full-thickness burn, for if there is no sensation present in the burnt area nerve-ending destruction is indicated. The burn also has a characteristic slatey grey or black colour. It is common for serious injuries to consist of a central full-thickness burn surrounded by areas of partial-thickness burns.

In the initial stages after a burn has occurred there will be marked swelling due to the release of fluid from the damaged tissue, known as oedema. In burns that involve the face and respiratory tract, this oedema may be life-threatening as it can lead to the occlusion of the airway. A further alarming development is that the patients' eyes may be closed by oedema, leading them to think that they have lost their sight. Inhaled gases, steam or even flames can cause serious damage deep down into the respiratory tract. Smoke can be highly dangerous due to the toxic nature of many substances used in modern furnishings, which when burnt release such highly toxic substances as cyanide and phosgene gas (Budassi and Barber, 1984). Many of the deaths that occur in fires are not due to burning, but more to asphyxiation by toxic fumes.

The combination of burn oedema and full-thickness, circumferential burns of the trunk or a limb is potentially disastrous. Full-thickness burns leave behind initially a tough, inelastic layer known as eschar, just as the tissue within the limb is trying to expand to accommodate the build-up of oedema. The result is a tourniquet effect and a rise in pressure that occludes the blood supply to the lower part of the limb. This will lead to loss of the limb due to gangrene unless the pressure is quickly released.

This should be done urgently by medical staff who perform an escharotomy, a longitudinal deep incision splitting the eschar and allowing expansion of deep tissue. No anaesthetic is needed as the nerve endings are dead.

In the past, burns affecting the hands were notoriously difficult to treat partly because of the time-consuming nature of dressings and bandages and also the problems of regaining mobility in the injured fingers. The modern approach has overcome these problems by the use of a plastic bag to enclose the whole hand, rather than traditional bandages (see below, p. 97).

The psychological aspect of burn injury should never be overlooked. The patient will have had a very frightening and painful experience, will still be in pain, and by the time the paramedic is on the scene his or her mind will have started to look to the future, wondering about scarring and disfigurement, and provoking great anxiety and fear. Consider also the parent of a burnt or scalded child who will have great feelings of guilt and blame with which to contend.

FIRST AID

Several simple steps to be taken immediately are of great value.

(1) Cold water, and lots of it, will greatly reduce the amount of damage that a burn can cause, so immerse the injured part in cold water or run cold water over it; this will give substantial pain relief, as well as reducing the severity of the burn injury.

(2) If the burn is due to a chemical agent, flood the affected area with continuous running cold water to dilute the burning agent and wash it away. Certain specific antidotes to some industrial chemicals are available. They should be prominently displayed and staff should be familiar with their use.

(3) If clothing is on fire, get the patient on the floor to protect his or her face, either put the flames out with cold water or smother them in a blanket, rug, coat or something similar. Smouldering items of clothing should be removed as they still contain heat, otherwise the area should be left alone because attempts to take clothes off may cause more pain and damage at this stage.

(4) If the burn is electrical, make sure the current is switched off before any further action. Use a brush with a wooden (*not* metal) handle or some similar object if necessary to separate the patient from the live source. Check for heart beat and breathing as cardiopulmonary resuscitation may be needed. Remember that electrical burns may be more extensive than they appear initially as the current may have penetrated deep within the limb causing severe damage to internal structures.

The golden rule for all burns, except for certain specific chemical burns where there is a special antidote, is never to apply any cream, lotion or other substance to the surface of the burn. This will contaminate the burn, increase the risk of infection, and only have to be removed immediately the patient reaches a medical facility. Either leave exposed and keep applying cold water, or dress loosely with a sterile dressing if one is available. Failing that, cling film makes an excellent dressing. If the patient feels thirsty, oral fluids are allowed in minor burns as surgery will not be needed and the body still needs to replace lost fluids.

PARAMEDIC AID

The basic principles of first aid still apply as outlined above; however, with the greater skills and equipment available the paramedic can do even more for the patient.

Assessment of Burns

As standard practice, start with an assessment. Find out what caused the burn and measure the surface area, how much pain the patient has, and how he or she is behaving. Check breathing if the face/neck area is involved, or if the patient has been in a smoke-filled area; is the breathing laboured or noisy? Look for evidence of soot or burns in the mouth and around the nose.

If there are respiratory problems give oxygen at once and monitor the respirations closely. Any suspicion of respiratory distress makes transfer to a medical facility of the highest priority where tracheostomy may be needed to keep the airway patent. Keep the patient sat upright to assist breathing.

Burn area is best measured using Wallace's rule of 9 (Fig. 5.2), which consists of dividing the body up into different sections which are multiples of 9% surface area. Count only those areas where there is significant burn, not just mild reddening of the skin as you might see in sunburn. Another useful fact to note is that the palm of the patient's hand is 1% of surface area. If the area is in excess of 15% shock will develop, it is therefore a matter of estimating how long it will take to get the patient to a medical facility; the sooner an intravenous infusion is started the better.

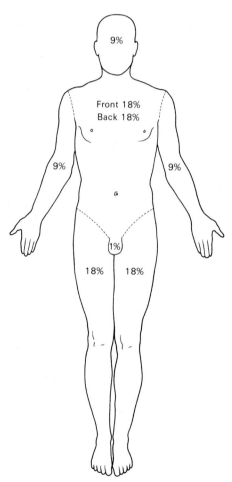

Fig. 5.2 Wallace's rule of 9 for estimating area of burns

The patient may not show signs of shock at first, but these will soon develop. If an intravenous infusion can be erected, then start off either normal saline (burns patients lose a great deal of sodium chloride) or Haemaccel. The larger the burn the quicker the rate of infusion needed, but the actual rate will depend on the area burnt and the patient's condition. *Caution*: do not become complacent as a patient who is initially in a good condition can deteriorate very quickly.

Oral Fluids

Settle (1974) describes the use of oral fluids in mass casualty situations. One such is Moyer's solution which consists of 4 g salt (sodium chloride) and 1.5 g sodium bicarbonate/litre, flavoured to disguise the salty taste. This solution can be achieved by mixing 1 litre of normal saline with 100 ml of isotonic sodium bicarbonate and 1 litre of tap water. Settle considers that this solution may be sufficient to ward off shock in cases of up to 30% burn. The use of oral fluids is not recommended in normal civilian practice; however, in remote locations or disasters where intravenous fluids are not available, they might be considered as a useful alternative. Great care should be taken in giving an oral salt solution due to the risk of vomiting, and the serious biochemical disturbances that can occur if too much is given.

Dressings

Every effort should be made to minimise contamination of the burn. Leave blisters intact as the fluid underneath is sterile, and concentrate on gently applying a non-adherent sterile dressing that can be well secured. Special prepacked sterile burn sheets are available. If there is a delay in moving the casualty, back the dressing with thick layers of gauze, as the burn wound will ooze a great deal of fluid very quickly and soak through a thin dressing. Once this has happened the dressing is no longer occlusive and bacteria have ready access to the burn. If a dressing *in situ* does become damp from burn fluid, do not remove it, but simply lay another dressing on top. The less the wound is handled the better.

Tissue Swelling

Swelling of tissue is very pronounced, so ensure that rings,

bracelets and any other potentially constricting items are removed as soon as possible. Elevation will help minimise swelling; this is particularly important when dealing with
full-thickness circumferential burns if you are to reduce the risk
of circulatory impairment.

Pain Relief

Pain relief can be achieved with the use of Entonox (see Appendix B, Fig. B.6). A surprising amount of relief can be obtained
from continual application of cold water. Even so patients will be
very frightened and anxious about their final appearance. As
has been discussed elsewhere (p. 56), the paramedic should be
honest and realistic about the long-term prognosis. It is simply
too early to say at this stage what the final cosmetic result will
be. Support should be offered, and also to relatives of the casualty, especially where the patient is a young child and the
mother is very upset and possibly feeling guilty.

Electrical Burns

If the burn is electrical, monitor the patient's heart rate during
transfer, as cardiac arrhythmias may be produced. Electrical
burns produce a very small surface area, but typically there may
be damage deep within the limb affecting nerves, tendons and
blood vessels. Elevate the limb (usually it is the hand or wrist
that is affected) and keep a close eye on circulation, sensation
and movement.

Hand Burns

Burnt hands can be left undressed if the transfer time is short, if
a delay is anticipated, they are best enclosed in a loose-fitting
plastic bag to prevent contamination, yet allow finger movement. Elevate the hand in a high arm sling to minimise swelling.

Checklist for Handling Burns

The handling of burns casualties can be summarised as follows:

(1) Remove the casualty from any immediate danger, check,
    the ABC of resuscitation.
(2) Employ first aid.

(3) Make a detailed burn assessment: cause, area, depth, pain, psychological state.
(4) Start an intravenous infusion if needed.
(5) Dress burn wounds, elevate limb, remove potential constrictions.
(6) Give psychological support.
(7) Transfer.

It should be noted that there is an upper limit to what is a survivable burn, dependent on the patient's age and general health. It is extremely unlikely that a young fit healthy adult will survive more than a 60% burn; even though they may look deceptively well when first seen by the paramedic, death will be within 12–18 h for such massive injuries.

References

Budassi S., Barber J. (1984) *Emergency Care*. St Louis: C. V. Mosby Co.
Sanders R. (1985) General treatment of burns. In Westaby S. (ed.). *Wound Care*. London: Heinemann.
Settle J. (1974) *Burns The First 48 Hours*. St Albans: SNP Ltd.

6. The Patient with Impaired Consciousness

INTRODUCTION

We have already considered the effects of head injury, and seen that the cardinal sign produced is a change in the level of consciousness. In this chapter we shift the emphasis to a group of serious medical conditions all of which manifest themselves by a reduced level of consciousness and constitute emergency situations requiring intervention from the paramedic.

DIABETES

In diabetes, the basic problem is that cells in the pancreas fail to make sufficient insulin, a hormone essential for the correct use of glucose by the body. The result is a build up in blood sugar levels that spark off a complex chain of events. The patient becomes very dehydrated, due to passing large amounts of urine (the body's way of trying to get rid of the excess sugar in the blood), there are serious disturbances in blood chemistry, and loss of consciousness. Brain damage may occur due to substances known as ketones which are formed by the faulty metabolism that occurs in this state.

Some people develop diabetes in later life, while others are diabetic from childhood. For many, their life depends upon self-injection of insulin and a carefully controlled diet, while other less severe cases manage by diet and tablets (such as glibenclamide) that augment their low pancreatic insulin production.

For people with diabetes to function normally, there needs to be a careful balance between dietary intake and insulin. However, if they forget their insulin or a meal, choose not to inject with insulin when they should, or develop an illness that throws extra stresses on the body (such as a cold), they may find that their blood sugar levels fall outside normal limits with serious consequences.

Many diabetics carry round with them a bracelet to inform anybody who finds them that they are diabetic. They may have appointment cards in their purse or wallet, or telltale sugar cubes to suck if they feel themselves going hypoglycaemic (too little sugar in the blood; see below). Further clues may be injection sites located over the abdomen, thigh or outer part of the arm. *These should not be confused with the injection sites of drug addicts* as theirs are located over veins, diabetics inject insulin subcutaneously (below the skin), *not* into a vein.

Hyperglycaemia

Hyperglycaemia is where there is too much sugar in the blood due usually to insufficient intake of insulin. The patient becomes drowsy and slides into a coma, the skin becomes very dry, the pulse is rapid and weak, blood pressure is low and the breathing sometimes is very deep and sighing in nature. A smell similar to pear drops may be detected on the patient's breath (due to the ketones).

A combination of these clues and the signs described above should suggest to the paramedic the likelihood that the collapsed patient is a diabetic in a hyperglycaemic state. It is now possible, however, to get a reasonable estimate of the patient's blood sugar level by widely used simple strip tests. The use of such test strips by ambulance crew would be a welcome step in developing advanced skills which should benefit patients. A drop of blood from the end of the finger or thumb is placed on a strip of plastic which has been chemically treated at the end. The blood reacts with the end of the strip and the resultant colour corresponds to the amount of sugar in the blood. A comparison chart is printed on the side of the strip container.

A random blood sugar in excess of 14 mmol/litre is taken as almost certainly indicating diabetes (Macleod, 1984) for diagnostic purposes in hospital tests. A reliable strip test is the BM Test Glycemie 1/44, which gives readings in various steps up to 44 mmol/litre. If the reading compares to the 11 or 17 mmol/litre steps, then diabetes is the likely cause of the patient's condition, and above that level the patient is almost certainly in a hyperglycaemic coma.

This is a real medical emergency that needs expert treatment as quickly as possible. The patient should be positioned and cared for as any other unconscious patient and rapidly transferred to a medical facility. An intravenous solution of normal saline, 1 litre, is required as quickly as possible to try to correct the patient's severe dehydration and sodium deficiency, followed by a second litre more slowly. A fast-acting insulin is also needed, but few patients have this type, rather they have a slow-acting form so that one injection will last for a period of many hours. If the patient cannot be speedily moved to a medical facility (for example owing to snowdrifts) every effort should be made to get the necessary fast-acting insulin and call a doctor to the patient.

Hypoglycaemia

The reverse of this situation is where patients have forgotten to have a meal after the insulin injection, resulting in blood sugar levels falling dangerously low. This tends to be the more common occurrence. Patients will become confused and drowsy, and behaviour may become quite odd and uncoordinated, so much so that they may be mistaken for being drunk. The pulse will be rapid and the skin may be quite sweaty, the telltale sign being a blood sugar of 2 mmol/litre or less when measured on a test strip. Diabetics usually know when they are going hypoglycaemic, and are taught always to carry round with them some sugar cubes so that if they feel themselves becoming lightheaded, they can suck a couple of cubes to try to get some glucose into their bloodstream quickly. Emergency personnel will encounter the hypoglycaemic situation with greater frequency in dealing with diabetics.

If patients are having a hypoglycaemic attack, try to persuade them to have a sweet drink or suck some sugar cubes if they can. Patients may be too confused to cooperate or may have lost consciousness altogether. In this situation a 50 ml intravenous injection of 50% glucose solution will usually restore patients to consciousness within a few minutes. If this treatment can be given at home, patients may not wish to attend hospital once revived. If the ambulance crew cannot cannulate a vein, an alternative treatment is to give an injection of glucagon, 1 mg i.m, which increases blood glucose levels by mobilising glycogen. This should be followed by the administration of dextrose by mouth as soon as the patient is able to cooperate.

Diabetic patients with dangerously low blood glucose levels can display some very odd behaviour and even be very aggressive. Always bear this in mind when called to a situation where a person is behaving oddly, with no smell of alcohol on their breath or other evidence of alcohol abuse. There are of course many possible explanations for such behaviour as we shall see later (p. 147), but one very mundane possibility is that the person is a diabetic with a blood sugar level that has fallen too low.

STROKES

A stroke is said to have happened when there has been a fault in the circulation of blood around the brain; either an artery has been blocked by fatty deposits (atheroma), or a clot (thrombus), or there has been a failure of the artery wall leading to a bleed. The effect can be very shortlived and minor or, at the other extreme, very quickly fatal.

As with head injury, the level of consciousness is often affected leading to either a period of confusion or unconsciousness. The part of the brain that controls movement may be affected, which in turn leads to a paralysis, usually affecting one side of the body. This is known as a *hemiplegia* and the patient will be seen to have lost the function of both arm and leg on the affected side, often together with facial muscles. Paradoxically the side of the body affected is always opposite from that part of the brain which has suffered damage. This is due to the fact that the motor nerves controlling movement cross over as they flow out of the base of the brain, so the left side of the brain controls the right side of the body, and vice versa. Speech may also be severely affected and, if the stroke affects the dominant hemisphere of the brain, may be lost altogether.

A stroke may be of sudden onset or develop more gradually. In the acute situation, vomiting often occurs. Incontinence of faeces and urine, due to complete relaxation of the sphincters, is likely if there has been unconsciousness. As strokes are a product of degenerative disease, they are most often found to affect the elderly, though middle-aged persons are also susceptible, especially if they are smokers and suffer from high blood pressure.

Assessment of Stroke

Stroke victims will often be elderly people who have lost the function of half their body, or at least developed severe weakness in the arm and leg. Consciousness may have been lost or impaired for a variable period of time, and they may still be unconscious, and possibly incontinent. Speech may be impaired. There may also be a history of fits after the patient's collapse.

There are many variations on this theme, however. There may have been a transient period of confusion and weakness which has now past leaving the person as normal. This passing phenomenon is called a *TIA, transient ischaemic attack*, and that is precisely what it is, a transient attack where there was a lack of blood to part of the brain (*ischaemia*).

Alternatively the stroke may affect the base of the brain. Here the picture is usually one of deep coma with extensor spasm upon painful stimulation of the limb. Hemiplegia is not usually present. Breathing takes upon a cyclical pattern known as *Cheyne-Stokes respirations*. There may be no apparent respiration for 10 s or more before the patient takes a series of deep breaths which gradually grow more and more shallow until they become imperceptible. This waxing and waning pattern of breathing is a serious sign in stroke victims. Hemiplegia is usually absent if a bleed has occurred on the surface of the brain below the arachnoid mater (see p. 42), logically known as a *subarachnoid haemorrhage*. Photophobia (dislike of the light) and neck stiffness are characteristic signs here.

After assessing patients and obtaining their history, the paramedic needs to transfer them to hospital. Ensure that the airway is clear (check especially for false teeth) and position them on their side. Take good care of the airway using suction and an oral airway as appropriate during transfer. Remember when lifting and moving patients that one side of the body may be paralysed, therefore they are unable to protect their limb from injury or to exert any grip. Ensure that limbs on the paralysed side are correctly positioned.

Patients who have suffered a hemiplegia may be totally unaware of the paralysed side of their body and of anything on that side of their body, including you. Talk to the patient from the unaffected side.

Loss of ability to speak will be extremely distressing, so be extra sensitive to this. The patient may still be able to communicate by responding to yes and no type questions by, for example, squeezing your hand once for yes and twice for no. The sudden loss of function and speech suffered by a stroke victim, plus the embarrassment of incontinence, all combine to make psychological support for both patient and family extremely important. Always assume that an apparently unconscious patient, can hear every word you say, whatever the cause of unconsciousness.

The long-term treatment of stroke victims is generally conservative. Many, however, make a good recovery, provided that they survive the initial stages of the illness. Good airway care and patient handling plus a smooth transfer to hospital are major contributions that the paramedic can make to the patient's long-term welfare.

FITS

When considering fits most people think immediately of epilepsy. There are in fact many reasons why a person may have a fit, and there are many sorts of fits. Fits are possible after head injury or a stroke, they may occur in states where blood chemistry is disordered due to diseases such as diabetes or kidney failure, or they may affect young children who are running a high temperature. A fit therefore does not have to be epileptic in nature.

Grand Mal Epilepsy

Having said that, let us first look at what normally happens in an epileptic grand mal convulsion or fit. A sudden electrical discharge in part of the brain is the cause of the fit. The patient may get a few seconds warning of what is to happen (the *aura*). The *tonic* stage comes first where the patient falls to the ground in severe muscle spasm, all the limbs are rigid, and due to the spasm not even the respiratory muscles are able to function, so the patient quickly becomes blue in the face and cyanosed. This lasts for about 20–30 s.

This is followed by the *clonic* stage, a period of generalised convulsion usually involving all four limbs and lasting 2 or so minutes. This gives way to a period of unconsciousness from which the patient gradually recovers, in a drowsy confused state at first, before regaining full consciousness.

It is usually in the *postictal* state, as it is known, that the paramedic first encounters patients who have had a fit. They are drowsy or unconscious, witnesses when questioned will describe a fit. Examination may reveal evidence such as a bracelet or anticonvulsive tablets (for example, phenytoin), of long-term epilepsy.

If patients actually have a fit while the paramedic is present, the correct procedure is to protect them from self-injury, and do nothing else. It may be very alarming to watch them turn blue or to see them thrashing around on the floor, but the advice remains the same, *do nothing*. Attempts to force an airway into the mouth will achieve nothing, and risk injury both to yourself and the patient. Let patients have their fit, while trying to remove any sharp or dangerous objects from the immediate vicinity. Try and protect the head if you can with a rolled up blanket, pillow or coat slipped underneath. The whole fit will be over within 2–3 min. If patients continue to fit, this is the rare condition known as status epilepticus, which requires urgent medical intervention with drug therapy to control it. Without such urgent intervention serious brain damage will occur, so there must be a rapid transfer to hospital, together with advance radio warning for the accident and emergency unit.

In the post-fit situation, care for the patient as you would any other unconscious or confused and drowsy patient. During the comatose period, incontinence may occur due to relaxation of muscle sphincters, which may subsequently be very embarrassing for the patient.

Patients may refuse to go to hospital on recovery, especially if they are confused. It is a wise precaution to try to persuade them to go with you. If this fails, consideration should be given to making sure there is a responsible adult to look after the patients until they are fully recovered, or contacting their general practitioner.

Fits can take many different forms from those described above, which is very much the textbook fit. However, the main principles remain the same: watch and observe, prevent patients from harming themselves during the fit by making their surroundings safe, and after the fit take good care of their airway, remembering that they may be unconscious for some while. Give oxygen in this immediate post-fit period and check for injuries, especially head injuries, that may have occurred during the fit. Remember that they may have bitten their tongue, causing bleeding in or out of their mouth.

HYPOTHERMIA

The effects of chilling the body below its normal temperature of 37°C may be seen in dealing with cases of exposure or in a more urban setting amongst the elderly. Hypothermia may be considered to start when the body core temperature has dropped below 35°C, and be very severe at temperatures of 30°C. Survival with a core temperature much below 30°C is very unlikely.

Exposure to Bad Weather

Exposure to bad weather is readily understood as a cause of hypothermia, the effect of wind chill greatly increasing the simple effect of the cold, a factor often overlooked by ill-equipped parties in mountainous areas. The wind chill factor, for example, produces a subarctic environment most of the year on the summits of the 900 m (3000 ft) Cumbrian fells, as the author knows only too well from personal experience!

Remember that temperature drops with altitude at the rate of about 1 °C per 165 m (550 ft), therefore still air temperatures in mountainous parts of the United Kingdom are going to be between 4 °C and 7 °C lower than the valleys. We are all familiar with the effect of a wind making it feel colder than it actually is. A 40 km/h (25 mph) wind will knock between 10 °C and 15 °C off the effective temperature that the body perceives or feels at typical UK temperatures. A reasonably pleasant April day in Keswick (temperature 10–14 °C; the upper 50s F), can therefore have effective temperatures below freezing on Great Gable a few kilometres away.

In the Elderly

Always consider hypothermia if called to the home of an elderly person who has not been seen for a period of time. It need not be bitterly cold for hypothermia to develop, as the ageing process affects the hypothalamus (that part of the brain which controls body temperature) as it can any other part of the body. Other social factors such as poverty, poor housing and heating added to lack of activity, and perhaps a tendency to confusion in some of the elderly, all contribute to increase the risks.

Effects of Hypothermia

The effect of hypothermia is to cause drowsiness, confusion and eventually coma if the temperature falls low enough (below 30 ° C). Shivering is seen in the early stages when the body temperature is in the 32–35 °C range. Serious disturbances of heart rhythm (cardiac arrhythmias) may occur in the low temperature range. An accurate estimate of the degree of hypothermia is obtained by taking a rectal temperature with a low-reading thermometer over a 7 min period. In the absence of a thermometer, you will be struck by how cold the person's skin feels, even in areas covered by clothing such as the abdomen. When dealing with hypothermia your hand tells you the patient has hypothermia, a thermometer just tells you how bad it is. If patients are comatose, they may even be mistaken for dead. Check carefully for a pulse or very shallow breathing; the pulse may be very feeble indeed.

Management of Hypothermia

As usual, the first need is to check the initial ABC of resuscitation and carry out any steps necessary, including giving oxygen via a mask. The body must clearly be reheated, but how? The answer is slowly and from within. There is no place for hot water bottles or other drastic remedies. If the periphery is warmed too quickly, this can be fatal as peripheral dilatation worsens shock; in addition, lactic acid which has been accumulating in the peripheries may be shunted back to the heart, leading to serious cardiac arrhythmias. The recommended method is to remove any wet clothing and place the patient in a space blanket, a highly reflective foil sheet that will gradually reheat the patient by reflecting the body's own heat back into the body. Make sure the patient's head is covered completely as a very large amount of heat is lost via this route due to the rich blood supply to the scalp.

Wrapped in a space blanket the patient will rewarm at between 0.5 °C and 1 °C/h, which is the desired rate. If possible heart rate should also be observed on an ECG monitor due to the risk of arrhythmias. The patient should be handled very gently and no exercise should be allowed as excess stimulation may provoke cardiac arrhythmias.

In persons who have been rescued from a cold environment, frostbite is also possible in addition to their hypothermia; this is due to the formation of ice crystals in the extracellular spaces within body tissue, resulting in severe damage and death of tissue. Typically the damaged area has a whitish appearance, and after initially giving rise to a slight burning pain or tingling feeling it loses sensation and feels numb. Swelling and oedema develop, and in late cases there may be gangrene.

The damaged area should be immobilised and protected from any further injury. Do not rub the area as this will cause further damage. Thawing out is an extremely painful process, and *on no account* should a patient use a limb that has thawed out. As the aim of care is to minimise the damaged area, try to prevent any further heat loss by, for example, removing any wet clothing and covering with dry blankets. Transfer as quickly as possible to a warm environment where the thawing out process can take place under controlled conditons with adequate pain relief.

When rescuing a person, always consider the effects of exposure to the environment as well as any obvious injury. Hypothermia can compound other injuries, and be a killer in its own right.

IMMERSION INJURY

The rescue of a person from water, be it fresh or salt, may present the paramedic with a dramatic situation. But there is more to this situation than drowning—the inhalation of water into the lungs.

Immersion in cold water has been shown to produce major cardiac arrhythmias. A common effect is to slow the heart rate down dramatically, the colder the water the slower the rate. People rescued from water may therefore at first appear to have no pulse as their heart may only be beating every few seconds. Respirations will also be very shallow and slow. The effect is one approaching a state of suspended animation, so resuscitation may be possible even in an apparently lifeless person who has been in the water a long time. There are well-documented cases of persons falling through ice into near-freezing water, being trapped under the ice for up to half an hour, yet being successfully resuscitated.

Management of the Drowning Patient

When confronted with a person rescued from drowning who is unconscious and who may at first sight appear dead, the important thing is not to give up. Clear the airway and start resuscitation. Feel very carefully for a pulse as it may be very weak and much slower than you have ever experienced before. Remember that chest compression carried out on a person whose heart is beating spontaneously is very dangerous. If possible, use a cardiac monitor to check for cardiac activity. Work on the patient for as long as it takes to get to the accident and emergency department. *The most surprising recoveries are possible in cases of apparent drowning.*

If the person is conscious when rescued, clear the airway as far as possible and transport him or her in an upright position, giving a high concentration of oxygen via a face mask. Pulmonary oedema is likely to develop in cases where water has been inhaled, so to assist breathing the patient needs to be in this upright position. In all cases of immersion, suspect hypothermia and treat accordingly if there is any evidence of this. The risk of developing pulmonary oedema means that even if the person appears to have made a good recovery, he or she should still be taken to hospital. Pulmonary oedema may happen up to 72 hours after the incident (secondary drowning).

Emergencies Through Deep Sea Diving

The paramedic may occasionally be confronted by an emergency that has arisen as a result of deep sea diving. This is a subject of great complexity, but the basic core of the problem is that, when diving, people subject their bodies to pressures greater than atmospheric, which in turn has significant physiological effects. For example, at a depth of only 10 m (33 ft), pressure is twice atmospheric and at 20 m (66 ft), three times atmospheric. This increased pressure in its turn will compress gas within the body, whether it be the lungs or hollow cavities such as the stomach, and will allow nitrogen to dissolve in the blood.

A rapid ascent without proper exhalation will result in the gas in the lungs expanding, leading to a rupture of the lung, spontaneous pneumothorax and the escape of bubbles of air into the circulation with potentially disastrous results (*air embolism*). If nitrogen has dissolved in the blood, a rapid ascent means there is not enough time for the gas to be reabsorbed, resulting in the formation of nitrogen bubbles in the blood (the '*bends*'). Compression of air in hollow body cavities leads to sharp cramping pains underwater (the '*squeeze*'), and panic may in turn cause too rapid an ascent.

Patients should be cared for in accordance with the basic ABC principles of resuscitation. They will need high concentration oxygen at a high rate of flow (10 litres/min). They should be placed in the left lateral position with the legs higher than the rest of the body, head down, to minimise the risk of brain damage due to air embolism. Urgent medical treatment is required for any pneumothorax that may be present, and decompression problems must be dealt with by recompression at a specialist unit. Emergency calls to victims of diving accidents should be treated with the greatest urgency, as serious injury can occur in only a few metres of water—as shown by the example quoted in Budassi and Barber (1984) of a pneumothorax occurring after diving only 1.2 m (4 ft). Remember also that in the UK water temperature is always going to be low, especially if the accident has occurred in a lake, as bottom temperatures all the year round will not be much above 4° C.

References

Budassi S., Barber J. (1984) *Emergency Care*. St Louis: C. V. Mosby Co.
Macleod J. (1984) *Davidson's Principles and Practice of Medicine*. Edinburgh: Churchill Livingstone.

7. Cardiac and Respiratory Emergencies

INTRODUCTION

The paramedic will often encounter serious emergency situations involving diseases of the chest. As the two principal systems that fill the chest consist of the heart and the lungs, it is not surprising to learn that these are most commonly the cause of the patient's distress.

CARDIAC EMERGENCIES

Note: Chapter 1 contained a discussion of what to do when the heart stops beating and resuscitation is needed. The reader is referred back to that chapter before proceeding with this next section.

The heart, like any other organ, needs a good blood supply to function. It is a muscular pump that has to beat some 70 to 80 times a minute for the whole of our life, and therefore needs a good blood supply delivered to its muscle, the myocardium, via the coronary arteries. If the blood supply to part of the myocardium is reduced, due to coronary artery disease, it will not be able to function efficiently. If on exertion the extra demand for oxygen cannot be met by the blood supply the result is pain, known as *angina*. This is similar to the cramp pain we have all experienced in the muscles of our legs when swimming or running too far.

If a *thrombus* (blood clot) lodges in a coronary artery, thereby completely blocking the blood supply to the myocardium, tissue death occurs. This is known as an *infarction*, hence the medical term *myocardial infarction* (MI), a very serious situation with a high risk of fatal arrhythmias developing, leading to cardiac arrest.

Myocardial Infarction

Patients with a myocardial infarction will usually experience severe, constant central chest pain of a gripping, vice-like quality (remember that the heart is situated approximately in the centre of the chest). Rest brings no relief, and the pain is often described as extending into the left arm or side of the face. Breathing may be rapid and the patient's colour pale. Cyanosis, not commonly seen, indicates that patients are in a grave condition. Patients are usually anxious and frightened, as if they know the seriousness of the condition. Blood pressure may be lower than normal, and in severe cases cardiogenic shock will develop (associated with cyanosis and a very poor survival rate). Many elderly patients may, however, have a myocardial infarction with few or any of these classic symptoms, simply collapsing and being short of breath (the silent coronary).

In view of the serious nature of the patient's condition, every effort should be made to stabilise the situation quickly (see p. 114) before transfer to hospital. The aim is to avoid further damage to the myocardium, and to resuscitate the patient if complications occur.

Myocardial damage can be limited by ensuring that the patients are completely at rest; do not allow them to walk to the ambulance, for example. Fear and anxiety will increase heart rate just when the heart needs rest, so you must therefore reassure the patient and provide a calm, confident environment. Relieve pain with Entonox (see Appendix B, Fig. B.6) as this also contains 50% oxygen which will increase the oxygen supply to the myocardium. If Entonox is not used, give the patient oxygen at 4 litres/min through a high concentration mask. It is vital that their damaged myocardium receives the best possible oxygen supply in order to minimise this damage.

The best pain relief is achieved by morphine or diamorphine given slowly, intravenously; but with the present controlled drugs regulations this must be administered by a doctor.

If the systolic blood pressure is below 100 or if the patient looks pale, it is best to transfer him or her lying flat. If cardiogenic shock is present—in other words, there is a systolic blood pressure of 80 or less accompanying a history suggestive of myocardial infarction—it is vital that you do *not* treat as for hypovolaemic shock and start running large amounts of intravenous fluid through. The problem is one of pump failure, not actual volume. Increasing the volume of fluid in the circulation will only make more work for the heart at a time when it is least able to pump effectively.

Attach patients to an ECG monitor and keep a close check on their rate and rhythm, remembering the pitfalls of monitoring discussed in Chapter 1. Explain carefully what you are doing and why to the patient and family in order to reduce stress and fear. Take a printed readout from the ECG machine, leads I,II and III, and label clearly with time, date, name, pulse and blood pressure at the time of recording.

A wise precaution is to secure an intravenous cannula. But the question of how many attempts to make to cannulate a vein is not always easy to answer. However, it may be very difficult to find a vein either because of the person's collapsed condition, or because they simply do not have very obvious veins. There are three dangers attached to continued attempts to set up a secure i.v. line: (a) you are using up precious time (see Fig. 1.12); (b) each attempt at setting up an intravenous infusion involves sticking a needle into the patient causing pain and distress; (c) each failed attempt makes it very difficult for that vein to be used again, making the hospital staff's job that much more difficult.

Securing an i.v. line may, however, be life-saving, because if the patient subsequently deteriorates you have an immediate route for giving vital drugs. Remember that the aim is not to give large volumes of fluid, rather to keep the cannula patent with a minimal flow rate. It also makes life a lot easier for medical staff in the accident and emergency unit if there is a secure intravenous route available. There are both advantages of securing an i.v. line, and disadvantages that follow from repeated attempts that fail. The good paramedic knows when to stop if first attempts have not been successful, and concentrate on moving the patient to hospital where more sophisticated facilities are available. The patient's clinical condition is always the determining factor, so do not be afraid to admit defeat when trying to establish an intravenous infusion.

In view of what has been said concerning stress and damage to the heart, the transfer to hospital needs to be carried out quietly and carefully. Klaxons, blue lights and sirens should not be needed. A speedy transfer is only required if the patient's condition deteriorates or is very poor to start off with.

Angina

Angina pain is usually associated with exertion and, like the pain of a myocardial infarction, will be located centrally in the chest, but unlike myocardial infarction will usually ease with rest. In addition the patient will often have glyceryl trinitrate tablets (GTN) to relieve the pain; these are usually placed under the tongue and sucked, but alternatively the drug may be applied as a paste to the chest wall. *Note:* Do not defibrillate on top of this paste. This drug is a potent vasodilator and works largely by reducing venous return to the heart and hence the work required from the left ventricle.

If a patient is taken ill with an attack of angina outdoors, you may be called to the scene. Although such attacks usually resolve without any further danger, it is mandatory to take all patients with central chest pain to hospital as a precaution. There is no clearcut dividing line between a bad episode of angina and a small myocardial infarction, as they tend to merge into one another.

A patient who suffers from angina may well have had a myocardial infarction, but through fear, self-denial, or simply not wanting to put others to trouble, may try and put the whole episode down to just another attack of angina and be very reluctant to go to hospital. Every effort should be made therefore to transfer the patient to a hospital accident and emergency department, even if there is reluctance to be admitted.

Heart Failure

Although there are many possible reasons why a person may be in a state of heart failure, the effect is broadly the same. The heart is no longer able to pump blood around the body efficiently and this in turn leads to the build-up of oedema (surplus tissue fluid). The body is effectively becoming waterlogged, and the lungs are the most likely vital part to be affected. The build-up of excess fluid in the lungs (pulmonary oedema) means that the exchange of gases that normally takes place in the lungs is inhibited and the patient is deprived of oxygen. Further, what oxygen is absorbed into the blood is no longer efficiently pumped around the body due to the failing heart.

The result is a patient acutely short of breath, very pale with rapid bubbly-sounding respirations who will be very distressed. Such patients are usually elderly, and the cause of their heart failure can be anything from an acute myocardial infarction to long-standing chest disease.

The aim should be to offer reassurance in what is a very frightening situation as the patient is fighting for breath. Keep the patient upright to aid breathing, and administer oxygen.

Some discussion is needed here about how much oxygen to give, a high or a low concentration. If patients have had long-standing respiratory disease (chronic bronchitis, for example), the mechanism that stimulates breathing will have altered. They will have got used to having a high carbon dioxide concentration in their blood (it is this CO_2 level that normally stimulates us to breathe), and so will rely on a low oxygen level to act as a respiratory stimulus. If they are given high concentration oxygen, the result will be an increase in blood oxygen levels to such an extent that the respiratory stimulus is lost and patients simply stop breathing.

Patients with a history of chronic respiratory disease (such as emphysema or bronchitis) should therefore only be given 24–28% oxygen via a controlled flow mask (Ventimask, for example). Other patients may safely be given 40% or thereabouts.

The transfer of patients to hospital should be rapid but with the minimum of fuss as stress will only exacerbate their problems. Intravenous drugs such as frusemide to get rid of the surplus body fluid can dramatically improve the patient's condition once in hospital. The medical staff will also wish to find the cause of the sudden episode of illness.

RESPIRATORY DISEASE AND THE EMERGENCY SITUATION

Respiratory emergencies by their very nature are very frightening experiences for the patient. Broadly speaking there can be two sorts of problem, either infection, leading to conditions such as pneumonia, or a mechanical problem.

Chest Infections

All ages may be affected by chest infections of varying degrees of seriousness. However, it is usually the very young and the very old who are most at jeopardy.

Shortness of breath is a common sign in chest infection, frequently associated with a temperature running above the normal 37 °C and a rapid pulse. Pain may also be present, but it is different from that in cardiac disease. The pain will increase on breathing in, unlike the constant pain of a myocardial infarction, or the angina pain that eases on rest.

In transferring patients to hospital keep them sat upright to aid breathing, and if they are in serious respiratory distress, administer oxygen via a face mask, high concentration if the acute emergency is *not* accompanied by a chronic condition. If flushed and feverish, avoid wrapping the patient up in blankets. Elderly patients seem prone to become confused when suffering from a chest infection, due to a lack of oxygen reaching the brain. Explain carefully where they are being taken and why.

Patients should be encouraged to cough if they feel like it; a sample of any material they manage to cough up, kept in a plastic container, will be of assistance to the medical staff on arrival at hospital.

Asthma

An acute asthmatic attack can be a very frightening experience for both the patient and family. Spasm of the muscle in the walls of the bronchial airways coupled with excess secretions causes extreme shortness of breath and gives rise to a feeling of great tightness across the chest. The patient cannot breathe out properly, in fact breathing becomes increasingly difficult, and there is a build-up of secretions that cannot be cleared by coughing. This blocks the smaller air passages and leaves areas of lung that can no longer be ventilated, adding further to the patient's distress. In some cases, deterioration may be rapid and death results.

Most chronic asthmatics carry with them an inhaler that administers a drug such as Ventolin, the effect of which is to relax muscle spasm in the bronchial airways, allowing normal breathing. However, to complicate matters an attack may not always be responsive to the inhaler, the patient may have forgotten it, or there may be a chest infection complicating the asthma. Attacks are therefore quite common for emergency personnel to deal with.

The patient will be acutely distressed, labouring to breathe and have a characteristic wheeze on breathing out. A history of asthma will usually be available, but try not to question the patient too much as speech will be very difficult. Try simple questions that can be answered yes or no by a shake of the head.

Medical aid should be summoned immediately or the patient transferred to hospital as quickly as possible as drug therapy is needed urgently to resolve the attack. Keep the patient sat upright, legs over the side of the trolley if requested, and administer high concentration oxygen (Macleod, 1984). Respiratory drive will not be affected, unlike the patient with chronic obstructive disease discussed on p. 116. Psychological support will be essential as an asthmatic attack is an extremely frightening experience for both family and patient. A useful tip to consider with an asthmatic child is gently squeezing the chest to assist expiration.

Pneumothorax

Problems associated with a pneumothorax have been discussed on p. 59. It is important to remember that a pneumothorax can also occur spontaneously without involving any trauma. It tends to occur among young adults, and is characterised by a rapid onset of breathlessness and pain or a feeling of tightness on the affected side of the chest which is made worse by breathing in deeply.

If the pneumothorax is of the type where a valve is formed from the lung into the pleura the patient may deteriorate very quickly, the so-called tension pneumothorax. Each time the patient breathes in, air enters the pleura, but cannot escape on breathing out. This build-up of air quickly collapses the lung and causes pressure to build up on the other lung. In severe cases the patient may become cyanosed, and emergency medical intervention is needed to save life (see p. 62).

Even if the picture is not as dramatic as this, the patient should be transferred to hospital quickly, and given respiratory support by means of upright positioning and high concentration oxygen via a face mask.

Pulmonary Embolism

This is a serious condition which may prove rapidly fatal. The cause of the problem is a thrombus plug which has been dislodged into the venous circulation. It will find its way to the heart via ever larger vessels and be pumped through a pulmonary artery to the lungs, where it lodges blocking the artery and cutting off the blood supply to the area of lung beyond. There is infarction of lung tissue, and if the embolism is large enough the patient may die.

The onset of symptoms is usually rapid and may closely resemble that of a myocardial infarction. The patient will be very short of breath and may be cyanosed; there may be haemoptysis (coughing up blood), and the blood pressure also falls. Death may occur within a few minutes, but Macleod (1984) points out that recovery is likely if the patient survives the first few hours.

Emergency personnel called to the scene of a collapse should proceed in the manner described for a cardiac arrest if the patient's heart has stopped beating. If the patient is still alive, treat as for a serious myocardial infarction, as it may not be possible to distinguish between the two conditions in the field and the same actions will be needed in either situation, but if an embolism is suspected move quickly to hospital.

Allergic Reactions

Serious allergic reactions may be fatal and they are included in this section because such reactions seriously impair the patient's breathing. A major part of the body's defence system involves the making of antibodies to neutralise any foreign protein (such as a virus). Exposure to the foreign material, or *antigen* as it is known, sets in motion a complex chain of events that leads to the formation of the desired antibodies. However, in some people, exposure to certain substances may produce a greatly exaggerated response that is pathological in nature. There is a sudden onset of oedema affecting the face and airway, and spasm of the bronchial muscles leading to serious respiratory distress. In severe cases there is a drop in blood pressure and shock develops. This latter situation is known as *anaphylactic shock*, and is usually caused by introduction of the offending material into the circulation via an insect sting, an injection, or ingestion of the allergen.

The patient will become very distressed and need great support. Rapid transfer to hospital is essential so the condition may be treated urgently with drug therapy (antihistamines, adrenaline and hydrocortisone). Administer high concentration oxygen via a face mask during transfer and keep the patient sitting up to assist breathing. In severe cases where the patient is collapsed this will not be possible, however, and full resuscitative measures will be needed. If necessary, summon medical aid to the scene. Speed is very much of the essence in dealing with a severe allergic reaction.

References

Macleod J. (1984) *Davidson's Principles and Practice of Medicine*. Edinburgh: Churchill Livingstone

8. Emergencies and Women

Although welcome changes are afoot to recruit women to the ambulance service, it is a fact that the majority of personnel are still men. It is important therefore for male personnel to understand that women have very real problems that are unique to them as women.

Crook (1985) has pointed out that female patients are still largely in the hands of male 'experts' who decide what is wrong with them and what is to be done for them. This has historically led to a false and distorted notion of women and their reaction to illness and pain: there are ideas that women are naturally always going to be weak and ill by the very nature of their bodies, alternatively it is asserted that their pain is hysterical, or psychological, or the result of some strange Freudian process of penis envy!

The crux of the matter is that men have defined illness for women, with the result that the dominant male role has been confirmed and reinforced over that of the 'weak' female. Thus childbirth is often seen as an illness, rather than a perfectly healthy and normal part of a woman's life. Consequent upon this has been the medicalisation of childbirth, leading to anxiety and fear upon the part of many a woman and ambulance crew when facing this most momentous occasion. For ambulance personnel the need is to see the woman in labour as a healthy person, who nevertheless may need some help in performing a perfectly normal function. Male staff should always remember that a woman's pain is real to her, and not be dismissive of 'another hysterical female'.

A fairly typical emergency situation involves an ambulance being called to a woman who has experienced severe lower abdominal pain, sometimes associated with vaginal bleeding. There are several possible causes varying from the relatively minor to life-threatening emergencies.

ABORTION

This term is used to describe the termination of pregnancy before the fetus is viable. According to Varma (1986), between 10 and 15% of pregnancies will end in a spontaneous abortion. It may be confused with an ectopic pregnancy (see p. 123) or delayed menstruation.

Classification

A common classification of abortion is as follows:

Threatened Abortion

This is an absence of menstruation (amenorrhoea) followed by slight vaginal bleeding. Pain is not usually a significant feature. The fetus is still viable.

Inevitable Abortion

Here there is heavy vaginal bleeding, followed by pain, which has been preceded by amenorrhoea. The fetus will be lost.

Complete Abortion

There is amenorrhoea followed by a variable amount of bleeding which has now stopped. The fetus is lost.

Incomplete Abortion

This is the usual outcome if abortion occurs before week 16 of the pregnancy. There will have been heavy bleeding and lower abdominal pain, and the patient may well have noticed the products of conception being passed with her blood loss.

Septic Abortion

This is an incomplete abortion complicated by infection of the uterine contents, commonly found after a criminal abortion. The patient will be pyrexial (38 °C plus), have a rapid pulse, marked lower abdominal pain, a purulent vaginal discharge and feel generally weak and unwell. This condition can lead rapidly to the development of septicaemic shock which carries a mortality rate of 30–50% (Varma, 1986).

Management

A threatened abortion is usually treated by bed rest. Psychological support is needed as the woman may have already lost a pregnancy and be very distressed at the thought of losing another. Ideally the family doctor should be called to deal with the patient at home, but if the woman is away from home at the time, a 999 call may bring you to the scene. In transferring a woman with a threatened abortion the important point to remember is to provide a reassuring, sympathetic environment.

If there has been heavy bleeding and pain, the situation is different as the pregnancy will be lost anyway. The woman needs admission for medical care and should be allowed nothing to eat or drink in case the gynaecologists decide that she needs immediate surgery. If she appears shocked, set up an intravenous infusion. Great psychological support is needed for the patient and her partner if present. Bleeding may be too heavy for a normal sanitary towel and the use of an incontinence pad may be indicated, a potentially embarrassing situation adding to her distressed state. The possibility should also be considered that the woman's family may not have known that she was pregnant, so respect her confidentiality at all times.

ECTOPIC PREGNANCY

An ectopic pregnancy occurs when a fertilised egg becomes implanted in a site other than the uterus, usually in one of the fallopian tubes. High risk factors in the patient's history are the use of either an IUCD (coil) or a progesterone-only pill for contraception, a previous history of pelvic inflammatory disease (PID) (such as salpingitis), previous gynaecological surgery, or a previous ectopic pregnancy. This latter fact increases the risk to between five and ten times above normal.

The patient is typically in her 20s and is complaining of cramping lower abdominal pain. Nausea and vomiting may be present and there will be a history of a missed period. If rupture occurs, then she may become critically ill, with heavy blood loss leading to the development of hypovolaemic shock and the need for emergency surgery. Varma (1986) estimates that 20% of patients where rupture occurs develop shock, and points out that 5% of maternal deaths are accounted for by ruptured ectopic pregnancies.

We are therefore dealing with a potentially life-threatening emergency that requires resuscitation following the principles laid down on p. 33. In addition, the patient will need a great deal of psychological support. Pain relief should be offered with Entonox (see Appendix B, Fig. B.6) and the patient kept nil by mouth as she will need surgery urgently. One fact to bear in mind is that approximately half the women who have suffered an ectopic pregnancy and undergone surgery are still capable of conceiving again. Your patient may find comfort in this fact.

MENSTRUAL DISORDERS

It might be thought that calling an ambulance for bad period pains is extremely unlikely, and if it did occur the person in question would be guilty of abusing the emergency ambulance service. Such a view is wrong on both counts! Calls are made to attend young women in great distress as a result of what, with the benefit of hindsight, turns out to be no more than a bad period. No male can know the feelings and sensations that accompany menstruation, and unless you are there at the time, you cannot appreciate the social circumstances surrounding the situation that may have led to a 999 call.

The following three aspects of menstrual disorder should be considered.

Menorrhagia

This is an extremely heavy flow of blood, or a menstrual flow over a prolonged period of 7 days or more. Varma (1986) reports this disorder as affecting between 5 and 10% of women. It is possible that the woman or family member may panic at the heavy loss and call an ambulance. It is important to find out if there had been a missed period as this would indicate the possibility of a pregnancy, and consequently the woman may be having an abortion. Such enquiries should always be carried out privately with the greatest discretion. You may get a very different answer from a young woman when her mother is within earshot than when she is alone.

Dysmenorrhoea

This is pain accompanying menstruation which may be so severe that 10% of women actually suffer incapacitation for between 1 and 3 days every month as a result (Varma 1986). It may be accompanied by a variety of other symptoms that can cloud the issue, such as nausea, vomiting, headache, dizziness and tiredness. It most commonly affects young women in their late teens or early twenties.

A common situation involves a woman being taken ill in a public place and a well-meaning member of the public dialling for an ambulance. The woman may be very distressed when you arrive, or alternatively just wanting all the fuss to go away. Tactful enquiry will often reveal a history of bad periods and she may well be able to confirm she has just started one. It is probably wise in such a situation to take her to hospital in any case as there is always the possibility of something more serious, for example acute appendicitis, being masked.

Premenstrual Syndrome

Premenstrual tension (PMT) can occur between 15 and 2 days before menstruation, although 4–10 days is the most common time. Varma (1986) estimates that between 30 and 40% of women suffer from symptoms to some degree, and that of these some 5% suffer severely incapacitating symptoms.

Symptoms vary from nervous tension, depression, anxiety, fatigue, dizziness and include a generalised bloated feeling, especially of the breasts and abdomen. These are real problems for the woman, and may contribute to a very distressed state. Male emergency personnel should not dismiss their patient as a 'typical neurotic female', but accept that she is suffering real problems needing help and understanding, and either call her own doctor or take her to hospital.

PREGNANCY AND TRAUMA

A pregnant woman may be the victim of trauma, either accidentally or deliberately. In the United Kingdom, blunt trauma is the most common form of injury; penetrating injury, associated usually with gunshot or knife wounds is rare.

Blunt trauma may lead to placental separation or uterine rupture, resulting in fetal death. The uterus acts as a shock-absorber for a pregnant woman, so many of the abdominal organs are protected from the worst effects of trauma. However, this is not true of the spleen and liver which become displaced and distended, making them more vulnerable to injury. Fractures involving the pelvis have serious implications for the pregnancy.

Assessment of a pregnant woman after trauma is more difficult as her pregnancy may mask vital signs. The increased blood volume associated with pregnancy means that hypotension and tachycardia may only become apparent when the woman has lost a third of her blood volume (Judd, 1985). Severe internal bleeding may therefore not be noticed until much later than in a non-pregnant patient. The woman's body reacts to shock by closing down blood supply to non-vital organs including the uterus, with potentially disastrous consequences for the fetus.

Positioning of the pregnant woman is very important. Place her in a left lateral position as this increases blood supply to the uterus. If she is left lying on her back for long period of time the weight of the uterus pressing on the vena cava will decrease venous return to the heart and therefore make shock worse. Both the woman, and her partner if present, will need a great deal of psychological support in transit to the accident and emergency department.

Complications of Pregnancy

Several serious conditions may develop during the course of a pregnancy which threaten the life of both mother and fetus.

Placenta Praevia

This occurs when part or all of the placenta covers the cervical os (the entrance to the uterus), leading to heavy *painless* bleeding and the development of shock. This condition is associated with the last 3 months of pregnancy and necessitates caesarean section as a matter of urgency. Treatment is as for shock, and psychological support and a rapid but smooth transfer to hospital are needed.

Abruptio Placentae

This condition involves the separation of the placenta from the uterine wall and occurs usually at about 20 weeks of gestation. The woman will suffer heavy, *painful* bleeding and be shocked. Fetal heart sounds will be absent if more than 50% of the placenta has separated, indicating death of the fetus.

Eclampsia

This toxic condition associated with seizures and fits can lead to a lack of oxygen in both the fetal brain as well as the mother's. The woman will be suffering from headaches, nausea and vomiting, and have a raised temperature and blood pressure (systolic above 140) in addition to fits. She should be given high concentration oxygen and transferred to hospital immediately, but carefully.

CHILDBIRTH

Health authorities have carefully laid down procedures for dealing with obstetric emergencies which must of course be adhered to at all times involving summoning the midwife or a 'flying squad' emergency team. However, Flint (1986) has written that a mother never forgets her midwife and it is a fact that sometimes the midwife is a member of the ambulance service. There are therefore many mothers with fond memories of the ambulance service!

A woman in labour may, for various reasons, not make it to the maternity hospital in time (the more babies a woman has had, the shorter her labour tends to be), leaving the ambulance crew to assist her in giving birth. Always ask about her previous pregnancies and whether there were any complications. Labour may be divided into the following three stages.

Stage 1: Dilatation Stage

Uterine contractures occur and the membranes rupture. Average length is about 12 h in a woman having her first baby, 7 h for a subsequent pregnancy. This period ends with the cervix completely dilated.

Stage 2: Expulsion Stage

This is from the full dilatation of the cervix through to the complete expulsion of the fetus. The mother is bearing down on her own and rarely needs any encouragement to push. Flint (1986) describes how most women know when and how to push their baby out and will adopt the position they find best, often standing with support or kneeling on all fours. The traditional medical position for delivery has been for the woman to be on her back with knees bent, a position that has fallen from favour with more progressive midwives who let the woman find her own position.

Signs that delivery is imminent include the passage of a large plug of bloody mucus, frequently occurring contractions, a bulging vulva and anus due to pressure from the baby's head as it descends and finally the sight of the baby's head itself beginning to emerge.

Stage 3: Placental Stage

This is the period of time between the birth and the expulsion of the placenta, usually 5–15 min.

To assist the mother in the delivery of her baby the fundamental requirement is to keep calm yourself. The environment should be warm, clean and private, although in an emergency situation this ideal may not always be achieved. Encourage the mother at all times and if possible put on a pair of sterile gloves.

When crowning has occurred (the whole of the top of the baby's head is first seen) exert a gentle pressure on the head to prevent too rapid an expulsion. Support the head with both hands and allow natural rotation of the baby to occur as it is pushed out.

During birth, check for the position of the umbilical cord and if it is around the neck slip it over the baby's head. If the cord becomes tangled tightly around the baby's neck at birth, severe brain damage may result as it cuts off the supply of oxygenated blood to the baby's brain. If it is wrapped around the neck and cannot be slipped free it must be cut immediately. This is done by clamping the cord in two places and cutting between the clamps, allowing its release. Using a mucus extractor suction should be gently applied to the nose and mouth of the infant to clear the airway. Newborn infants are nose breathers so the nose must be cleared first. It is then a matter of guiding the infant's shoulders as the rest of the birth is completed before finally wiping the eyes clear of amniotic fluid with cottonwool balls.

Further gentle suction, holding the infant's head down, should be carried out at once and at this stage spontaneous breathing should occur. The baby may be laid face down on your knees and the feet elevated while the chest is gently massaged to help clear the airway. If breathing still does not occur stimulate the baby by further gentle massage. Failure to breathe at this stage indicates the need for cardiopulmonary resuscitation.

There is no rush to cut the cord. Wait until it has stopped pulsating then clamp it in two places about 15–25 cm (6–10 in) from the baby and cut between the clamps with sterile scissors if possible.

The infant should be kept warm by wrapping in a blanket and presented to the mother as soon as possible. Let her see all that is going on; it is her baby after all.

The delivery of the placenta is heralded by the umbilical cord advancing 5–7.5 cm (2–3 in) further out of the vagina and a large rush of blood. Ask the mother to bear down and holding the cord yourself, apply a gentle traction but do not pull the cord. Massaging the uterus will assist delivery. The placenta should be saved in a basin as it may be needed for examination later.

After the Birth

When birth is complete it is a matter of caring for the mother by cleaning her and making her comfortable while keeping a close watch on the baby's breathing and colour. Some bleeding will occur, 250–300 ml is normal after delivery. However a heavy bleed of more than 750 ml is possible and constitutes a post-partum haemorrhage which will lead to shock. Apart from the normal resuscitative measures, Budassi and Barber (1984) recommend that the paramedic should also massage the uterus and insert a fist into the vagina to try to control the bleeding.

In most cases the birth will be uncomplicated. However, there are possible problems of which the most serious are either a breech delivery or prolapsed cord. In the case of a breech, the fetus presents either buttocks or feet first. This is dangerous as there is a greater risk of à prolapsed cord or of the fetus inhaling amniotic fluid. The legs or buttocks should be supported and the protruding part gently pulled out with the back upwards. Bring the arms out and deliver the head by placing a finger in the baby's mouth to flex the head while pulling on the shoulders. If the head is not delivered in 2 min apply firmer pressure and have a second person press on the mother in the suprapubic area.

If the cord is prolapsed it will precede the infant. Fetal heart tones will be decreased indicating fetal distress. The mother should be given high concentration oxygen via a mask to help oxygenate the fetus. A gloved hand should be inserted with the aim of elevating the fetal head slightly, thereby relieving pressure on the cord. Both hand and cord should be left where they are; do not attempt to place it back in the vagina. Alternatively, the woman could be placed kneeling with her knees up to her chest and her head down—the genupectoral position. Provided that you can feel pulsations in the cord and the fetal head is held in this position, a supply of oxygenated blood should continue to reach the fetus. An immediate caesarean section is required, so urgent transfer to the maternity hospital is indicated.

Reactions to Childbirth

A woman's reaction to childbirth can vary enormously. As Flint (1986) has stated: 'Birth is remembered by the woman for ever. It colours her feelings about herself, about her baby and about the rest of her family.... Giving birth can be an ecstatic and miraculous experience for a woman, but it can also be a nightmare.' Lucky is the ambulance crew who can assist a woman in this ultimate celebration of life. And yet, it is not always this way. The woman may not react in quite the way you would predict. Webb

(1985) has shown that the existence of a so-called 'maternal instinct' is very questionable, and that many women do not react in the expected way after birth.

STILLBIRTH AND NEONATAL DEATH

Sometimes the pregnancy does not go to term, and the infant dies in the uterus or at birth. Flint (1986) describes how important it is for the parents to have the chance to see and hold their baby, even though it is dead. They may not want to touch the dead infant, but they should be given the opportunity to do so. The parents have the full grieving process to work through, all the more difficult for a child they never knew, or whose life was measured in minutes rather than years. Even if the infant is handicapped, let the mother see it, for nothing will be as bad as she will imagine it to have been in the weeks and months that lie ahead. This is obviously a very emotional time for all concerned, including the ambulance crew. Your support and comfort will be appreciated for the rest of the woman's life.

References

Budassi S., Barber J. (1984) *Emergency Care*. St Louis: C. V. Mosby Co.

Crook J. (1985) Women in pain. In Copp L. A. (ed.) *Perspectives in Pain*. Edinburgh: Churchill Livingstone.

Flint C. (1986) *Sensitive Midwifery*. London: Heinemann.

Judd M. (1985) Women's health problems, in accident and emergency. In Walsh M. (ed.) *Accident and Emergency Nursing, A New Approach*. London: Heinemann.

Varma T. R. (1986) *Manual of Gynaecology*. Edinburgh: Churchill Livingstone.

Webb C. (1985) *Sexuality, Nursing and Health*. Chichester: John Wiley and Sons.

9. Infectious Conditions

Infectious diseases come in varying degrees of severity, ranging from the common cold through to AIDS. Unfortunately, without even being aware of it you may be handling patients in the field who have infectious conditions. Basic precautions should therefore be taken at all times.

Each authority will have its own procedures for transporting patients with infectious diseases; it is your responsibility to make sure you are familiar with them and adhere to them at all times. They will be concerned with: removal of all non-essential equipment from the vehicle; protective clothing for crew; and disinfection procedures after completing the transfer. Failure to follow these procedures may endanger both you and your patients.

Emergency personnel should remember that while an infected patient *may* show signs of disease, he or she may also be carrying an organism without actually showing any clinical evidence of suffering from the relevant disease. Hepatitis B is one well-known example of this phenomenon. This further underlines the need for caution by emergency personnel.

HEPATITIS

Two principal forms of hepatitis are recognised: A and B. Hepatitis A, is caused by a virus found in the gut, which primarily attacks the liver, and may be spread by faecal contamination or droplet infection; it can be fatal. Hepatitis B lives in the blood stream and its spread is therefore associated with contaminated blood products and needles, accidental injection, infection via uncovered wounds, or sexual intercourse.

Personal hygiene and following the correct procedures offer the best protection in dealing with possible hepatitis infection: wash your hands thoroughly after handling any materials that have been contaminated with body excreta; ensure that any wounds or scratches on your hands are protected by sticking plaster; when inserting intravenous cannulae or giving an injection, be careful not to prick yourself with the cannula or needle; always try to avoid contaminating yourself with the patient's blood. An increased use of disposable gloves would be a welcome development, as even situations such as childbirth may expose personnel to bloodborne infectious diseases.

Both forms of hepatitis have lengthy incubation periods, 15–45 days for type A and 30–100 days for type B. Immunisation is available, although the policy on its availability varies between health authorities. Remember that infection can occur through even the smallest cut associated with, for example, a piece of windscreen glass or an accidental prick with a needle. If there is any doubt, the matter should be reported to a senior officer immediately as vaccination after exposure must be carried out within 48 h.

AIDS (ACQUIRED IMMUNE DEFICIENCY SYNDROME)

Regrettably AIDS has been the subject of much hysterical, sensational and totally unfounded speculation in the popular media. It is a bloodborne disease found amongst intravenous drug abusers, haemophiliacs (due to the use of contaminated blood products), and as it is also sexually transmitted, it may be found amongst persons of either sex who are sexually active, although the majority of victims currently are homosexual or bisexual. At present there is no cure and death seems inevitable as the disease destroys the body's natural defence mechanism against infection.

Meanwhile, emergency personnel should ignore the hysteria

generated in the popular press and concentrate on medical facts and the procedures outlined in the section on hepatitis (p. 132). Controversy surrounds the risks of mouth-to-mouth resuscitation, therefore it should be noted that there is *no medical evidence* to suggest that AIDS is passed on by kissing or oral secretions. It is a hypothetical risk anyway, as personnel would in practice always use a bag/mask system or Brooks airway. Refusal to administer mouth-to-mouth resuscitation if you do not have advanced equipment is a matter between you and your conscience. If you do not, the person will certainly die, if you do, the risk is no greater than kissing someone. A person suffering from AIDS is a human being like anybody else, they are just going to die sooner, that is all. They therefore deserve the highest standard of professional care that you can offer.

CHICKENPOX, MEASLES AND OTHER CHILDHOOD DISEASES

Chickenpox and measles are but two examples of common infectious diseases of childhood, both due to virus infection. Most children come through these illnesses without requiring hospitalisation, although complications may occasionally lead to admission. Immunity is acquired once a person has had the disease, therefore most emergency personnel should not be unduly worried about transporting cases assuming they have had chickenpox or measles as children. Measles is passed on by droplet infection, that is, by the fine spray associated with sneezing, talking or just breathing out, while chickenpox requires contact with the infected skin eruptions that are characteristic of the illness.

INFLUENZA

Influenza is also caused by a virus, but one that has many mutations and forms with the result that although we may suffer an attack and acquire immunity to that particular strain, we may later be exposed to a different strain to which we have no immunity. The common cold and influenza are spread by droplet infection, so it is possible for patients to infect crew and vice versa. Ambulance personnel who report for duty suffering from the effects of a heavy cold or influenza are not therefore doing their patients or their colleagues any favours as they may then pass on that infection very easily. In the case of very young children and the elderly the implications of influenza or a severe chest infection secondary to a bad cold are very serious indeed, possibly fatal.

TUBERCULOSIS

Formerly a much-feared illness, and with good cause, it is still with us today, particularly among poor immigrants, the elderly and the worst-off in our society. Healthy adults will, however, have acquired sufficient natural immunity to tuberculosis to make it very unlikely that they would be infected by a patient. However, if a patient is found to be suffering from the active form of the disease, arrangements should be made via a senior officer to check the paramedic's immunity status and to check that vaccination is available if necessary.

FLEAS AND LICE

Infestation is possible, especially amongst those who have neglected themselves, such as vagrants. Avoid close contact as much as possible, have a good shower back at the station and change your clothing, which may need placing in a separate bag for disinfestation, depending on local procedures. The ambulance may likewise need fumigation. The next patient you carry will appreciate your observation of correct procedure!

FOOD POISONING AND SALMONELLA INFECTIONS

The salmonella organism has many strains that can cause different conditions. In the United Kingdom we are most familiar with food poisoning as the end-product of salmonella infection, although in regions where hygiene is poor typhoid and paratyphoid are common. The manner of infection is via the faecal–oral route usually due to contamination of a water supply by human excreta. As the incubation period is 10–14 days, it is possible for persons to contract typhoid overseas, and return to the United Kingdom before developing the full symptoms of the illness. Apart from fever and general malaise, diarrhoea is a striking feature of the illness.

The commonly seen condition of food poisoning is associated with diarrhoea and vomiting which develops within 48 h of eating infected food. The salmonella group of bacteria are usually to blame, and modern methods of factory farming and deep freezing contribute heavily to the spread and transmission of disease, especially via poultry. Dysentery is usually caused by the shigella genus of bacteria, and the most common form of spread is via unwashed hands after defaecation. Epidemic conditions occur in crowded populations with poor sanitation, as contaminated food and flies add to the transmission of the disease.

In cases of diarrhoea and vomiting, food poisoning should be high on your list of possible causes. Find out what the patient has eaten recently and if others shared the same meal. What is their condition? Treat any faeces as potentially infective, wear gloves, and pay great attention to handwashing.

EXOTIC FEVERS

Rabies

Man is most frequently infected by dogs, but infection via other animals is also possible. Inoculation with the virus is needed to contract the disease, hence biting is the usual cause. Symptoms usually appear with 4–8 weeks and the chances of survival in established cases is very small. If vigorous treatment is commenced within 48 h of biting, including thorough toilet and debridement of the wound, and the administration of antirabies serum, survival is possible.

Lassa Fever

Outbreaks have occurred in West Africa, the virus being transmitted in the urine of the multimammate rat. Macleod (1984) reports that human-to-human transmission is possible via direct inoculation and possibly inhalation. Great care is therefore needed in dealing with the patient's body fluids. Mortality rates vary between 36% and 52% (Macleod, 1984). The diagnosis should be considered in any person who has become generally unwell within 10 days of leaving West Africa.

Ebola Fever

The virus responsible for this disease is identical to that which caused an outbreak of the so-called Marburg fever (otherwise known as green monkey disease). The natural reservoirs in Uganda, Sudan and Zaire have all been seen as the origins of these viruses. An incubation period of 5–9 days leads on to an acute fever which has a high mortality rate. The mode of spread of the virus is unknown.

The possibility that you may be dealing with a rare and virulent disease should always be at the back of your mind, and as such encourage you to observe good hygienic practice at all times and adhere closely to agreed procedures. If you did find yourself with a person on board who might be suffering from one of these rare diseases, extra precautions are necessary. Notify control at once, and stay inside the vehicle, even if you break down, until the appropriate precautions can be taken to receive and isolate the patient safely. In effect, you have to be prepared to put yourselves, the patient and your vehicle in a self-imposed quarantine.

PSYCHOLOGICAL STRESS

One final comment should be made concerning the psychological stress imposed on a patient if they are greeted by ambulance crew dressed up in disposable white suits, masks and gloves. This is likely to be extremely distressing leading to feelings of isolation, alienation and impending death. However, emergency personnel need to protect themselves and their subsequent patients. Local policy should therefore be adhered to in connection with protective clothing at all times, but that policy should also be sensitive to the psychological needs of the patient.

References

Macleod J. (1984) *Davidson's Principles and Practice of Medicine.* Edinburgh: Churchill Livingstone.

10. Radiation Casualties

INTRODUCTION

We live today in a nuclear age; consequently emergency personnel must be familiar with the potential hazards that surround the nuclear industry, both peaceful and military. Major accidents involving nuclear materials have fortunately been very few and far between; however incidents at Three Mile Island (in the United States), BNFL Sellafield (in the United Kingdom), and most recently Chernobyl (in the USSR) demonstrate that no system is foolproof. Accidents it seems will always happen, and it is the job of the emergency services to pick up the pieces afterwards.

BASIC PHYSICS AND RADIATION

It is important first of all to understand the basic physics of radioactive materials and ionising radiation. A simple model of the atom postulates that there is a *nucleus*, a central core of positively charged particles (protons), and particles carrying no charge (neutrons). This nucleus is surrounded by a cloud of much lighter negatively charged particles, called electrons, which have about 1/2000th of the mass of one proton or neutron. The number of negatively charged electrons equals the number of positively charged protons, therefore an atom is normally electrically neutral.

The chemistry of an element is defined by the number of electrons orbiting the nucleus; this varies from 1 for the lightest element of all, hydrogen, through to 92 for the heaviest naturally occurring element, uranium.

Atoms are held together by various forces, usually in a stable form. Contained within the atom, or to be more precise the nucleus, is a tremendous amount of energy. Two aspects of this simple model of atoms are of interest to us here. First, not all forms of elements are stable; some are unstable and will gradually decay emitting subatomic particles and packages of energy as they do so. The rate of decay is variable and is measured by the half-life, which simply means the amount of time it takes for half of a given mass of the element to decay. This can vary from fractions of a second to millions of years. Such elements are said to be *radioactive*.

Second, the emitted particles or packages of energy are capable of causing changes within other atoms that they encounter. Such emissions are called radiation, and when they are capable of causing changes within other atoms they are known as ionising radiation. *Ionisation* is the term given to this process of change within the atom due to outside radiation.

Ionising Radiation

As ambulance staff, we are most concerned with what happens when such ionising radiation strikes the human body and the changes it leads to within living tissue. These changes most affect cell division and, as we shall see later, it is the most rapidly dividing cells in the body that are most vulnerable to ionising radiation.

Ionising radiation can take different forms, as shown in Table 10.1, which also indicates that different forms of radiation have different penetrative powers. It is the amount of energy imparted to the human body by the radiation that is crucial, as the more energy we absorb the greater the damage (just as a punch on the jaw from Frank Bruno will be more damaging than a gentle pat on the cheek from your local accident and emergency department sister!). The amount of energy in radiation used to be measured in rads, but new units are grays, 1 gray (Gy) = 100 rad. The amount of energy absorbed by the human body was measured in rems, the new units being sieverts (Sv), 1 sievert = 100 rem. For practical purposes, in many situations 1 rad = 1

Table 10.1 Common Forms of Ionising Radiation

Radiation type	Nature of radiation	Penetrating power air	body tissue
Alpha (α)-ray	Particle stream, each particle consists of two protons, and two neutrons	6 cm	< 1 mm
Beta (β)-ray	Stream of electrons	5 m	< 2 cm
X-rays	Energy released by electrons changing position in atom	10–100 m	whole body
Gamma (γ)-rays*	Energy released by nuclear particles reorganising position	100+ m	whole body
Neutrons*	Stream of neutrons	100+ m	whole body

* The penetrating power of γ-rays and neutrons is such as to make wearing lead aprons as used for radiology of little use.

rem. Table 10.2 summarises the effects of exposure to ionising radiation of different energy levels.

People are said to be *contaminated* if they still have radioactive material on their body, such as dust or debris, that is radioactive after an accident and is emitting ionising radiation that will affect others as well as themselves. However, when people have been *irradiated* the stream of ionising radiation has passed through them; the damage has been done, but they are not radioactive and therefore no danger to anybody else.

HOW RADIATION ACCIDENTS MAY OCCUR

Let us now look at some possible scenarios for radiation accidents. First, there is the possibility of a transit accident; many

Table 10.2 Effects of Radiation—Radiation Sickness Syndrome

Whole body acute radiation (exposure in cGy)	Effects
0–150	Either no symptoms or generally unwell and nauseated; significant fall in blood lymphocyte count
150–400	Bone marrow disease. Days 1–2 after exposure: unwell, nausea and vomiting. Weeks 2–3: fever, skin haemorrhages, mouth ulcers, loss of hair at more than 300 cGy. Marked fall in blood count with maximum bone marrow depression at 30 days
400–1000	Enteric disease. Day 1: unwell, nausea and vomiting. Weeks 1–2: fever, profuse bloody diarrhoea, loss of gut lining. Week 3: bone marrow disease if still alive. At 400–450 cGy, 50% mortality for young fit adults; at 600 cGy, near 100% mortality
1000 plus	Central nervous system disease; lethargy, unsteadiness, convulsions, coma and death within days
4000 plus	Death in a matter of hours

Based on data in BMA (1983), and after Hartog, Humphreys and Middleton (1981).

journeys are made each year to carry radioactive materials, varying from small amounts for laboratory and industrial purposes through to the large and highly radioactive flasks of material that are moved from nuclear power stations to BNFL Sellafield for reprocessing. Significant quantities of nuclear military hardware are also moved around the United Kingdom on the road network. Accidents may also occur at a nuclear power station, laboratory or military installation. Radioactive materials are also widely used in industry and hospitals. It is likely, therefore, that throughout the country there is the possibility of an accident involving radiation.

The situation may have several possibilities, with the number of casualties varying from one or two to possibly millions. Casualties may have suffered no trauma, other than exposure to radiation (irradiated); or they may have been contaminated with radioactive material and therefore still be radioactive. Contamination may be on the surface of the body, hair, clothes etc., or they may have inhaled or swallowed radioactive material.

Alternatively, casualties may have suffered conventional trauma ranging from fractures, head and chest injuries, burns etc., and additionally been exposed to radiation (irradiated or contaminated). It is also possible that they may *think* they have been exposed to radiation when in fact they have not, and there is no immediate way of telling. Generally speaking, exposure to radiation makes the prognosis for conventional injury much worse, in addition to the effects of the radiation injury itself.

Emergency personnel face a dilemma at the scene of a nuclear accident. On the one hand they want to get to the casualties as quickly as possible, but on the other hand radiation is a significant hazard. Further, unlike fire or traffic on a motorway, this is a hazard you cannot see, smell, hear, taste or touch, so how do you know it is there, and how do you know your precautions are effective?

Following the Rules

At the scene it is vital that you follow the directions of radiation monitors, experienced personnel with measuring equipment that can measure radiation levels in the area and also the Fire Brigade. Protective clothing will prevent you becoming contaminated with radioactive material, but it will not protect you from ionising radiation (see Table 10.1). The situation may therefore arise where casualties will be left where they lie, radiation levels being too high for rescue staff to reach them. You may not absorb an immediately life-threatening dose by such attempts, but you will expose yourself to the long-term effects of radiation such as sterility and cancer.

Smith and Smith (1981) point out that there is no such thing as a safe dose of radiation; lower doses carry lower risks, but the risks are still there. The rate of development of cancer has been calculated at about 1–2 cases per 10 000 persons exposed per rad. Entry into an area where you may absorb 20 rad therefore gives you a cancer risk of between 1 in 250 and 1 in 500. Evidence from the Hiroshima and Nagasaki victims indicates that those who were exposed to 450 rad and survived subsequently developed cancer at a rate 25–50% above the natural frequency (Smith and Smith, 1981).

Statistics such as these must be borne in mind when dealing with radiation accidents. Emergency personnel must consider their own safety at all times, in addition to the casualties they are trying to assist.

Once a casualty has been rescued, resuscitation should be carried out in the normal way. This must take priority over decontamination, otherwise you will have nothing but a decontaminated corpse to show for your efforts. Removal of the casualty's clothes will probably accomplish 90% decontamination; after seeing to resuscitation priorities, this should be carried out before transferring the person to hospital.

Nuclear power stations carry stocks of iodine tablets for use in an emergency. Such is the physics of a nuclear reactor, that if there were an accident one of the radioactive elements that would probably be released is a form of iodine. The effect on the body is to increase greatly the long-term risk of cancer of the thyroid due to the fact that this organ stores and concentrates iodine naturally. The theory behind giving iodine tablets is that the body will preferentially store the safe form of iodine given in the tablets rather than the radioactive form, thereby reducing the risks. So if you are involved in a nuclear power station accident make sure you take advantage of the iodine tablet you will be offered.

The only other precaution you can sensibly take with radiation is to avoid it. Radiation intensity decays in accordance with the inverse square law; this means that whatever the radiation levels are to start off with, if you double the distance between yourself and the source, the intensity of radiation will be reduced by one-quarter. Keep as far away from any source of radiation as you can. Further, try to get as much solid material such as concrete between you and that source, as it will absorb considerable amounts of radiation.

NUCLEAR EXPLOSIONS

So far we have discussed civilian accidents such as might happen at a nuclear power station. It remains to consider what would happen in the event of a nuclear explosion. Chernobyl, it will be recalled, was a conventional explosion in 1986 apparently involving hydrogen and steam, which threw large amounts of radioactive material into the atmosphere. By comparison, the effects of a nuclear weapon detonating are awesome in the extreme.

To get some idea of the forces involved, it is estimated (BMA, 1983) that a medium-sized, airburst, 1 megatonne weapon would inflict fatal blast injuries on 98% of those within 4 km (2½ miles) of the point of explosion. There would be a zone 14 km (9 miles) in diameter in which 50% of the population would die, 40% would suffer serious injuries, and most normal buildings would be destroyed. In the 11 km (6½ miles) beyond this zone, a third of the population would suffer serious injuries from the effects of blast. Add to this the prediction that as far away as 12–13 km (about 7½—8 miles) the heat generated by the explosion would be capable of inflicting fatal partial thickness burns, and the scale of the problem becomes apparent.

Translating these sort of figures into a real example, the Royal College of Nursing (1983) showed that if a 1 megatonne weapon detonated over the centre of Bristol, there would be some 200 000 fatalities and 100 000 injured survivors. About 100 hospital beds would survive on the outskirts of the city, some 325 nurses and a few score doctors might escape uninjured. Ambulance personnel would fare no better.

It is small wonder that the BMA and RCN both concluded independently that the effects of one single nuclear explosion would totally overwhelm the NHS. It is also apparent that civil defence planning for a nuclear war is the utmost folly, yet plans involving the ambulance service are being actively drawn up. Emergency personnel have better things to occupy their time with than these fallacies. The Joint Legislative Forum on Nuclear War Preparedness in California has been told by State Director of Health, B.A. Myers (1982), that to plan for a hoax is a disservice to the people. The same comment applies in the United Kingdom, as the notion of surviving a nuclear war is the cruellest hoax of all.

CHECKLIST FOR STEPS TO BE TAKEN
AT A NUCLEAR ACCIDENT

These may be summarised as follows:

(1) Park the ambulance upwind, notify Control, approach with caution.

(2) Work under the direction of the incident officer or radiation control monitors *at all times.*

(3) Wear any protective clothing issued and take an iodine tablet.

(4) Treat casualties in normal way.

(5) Leave any clothes removed from casualties at the scene, *clearly labelled as contaminated,* in an appropriate area set aside for them.

(6) Ensure that you know which hospital is to receive the casualties and via which department; special arrangements may have been made to avoid the main accident and emergency department and use other facilities.

(7) Notify control when leaving the scene and check if any special route is to be followed.

(8) When transfer complete, notify the liaison officer. At all times remember that three factors protect you against radiation: (a) time, the shorter the time you are exposed the better; (b) distance, doubling the distance reduces the intensity of radiation to one-quarter of its intensity; (c) concrete shielding.

References

BMA (1983) *The Medical Effects of Nuclear War.* London: BMA.

Hartog M., Humphrey J., Middleton H. (1981) *Medical Consequences of the Effects of Nuclear Weapons.* Cambridge: Medical Campaign Against Nuclear Weapons.

Myers B. A. (1982) Editorial, *Journal of Public Health Policy,* June.

Royal College of Nursing (1983) *Nuclear War Civil Defence Planning, The Implications for Nursing.* London: Royal College of Nursing.

Smith J., Smith A. (1981) Long term effects of radiation. *British Medical Journal,* **283**, 3.

11. Psychological Aspects and the Emergency Patient

INTRODUCTION

Psychology is a vast field covering many aspects of human behaviour. How do we think and remember? How do we learn? Where do emotions come from? How do we perceive and understand the world around us? These are just some of the questions to which the study of psychology addresses itself.

It has become increasingly recognised that these areas have great significance for the care of the injured or acutely ill person. Walsh (1985) has already described the significance of these factors in the care of patients within the accident and emergency unit, and it can be seen that they are of equal if not greater importance in the prehospital situation. Paramedics will therefore benefit both themselves and their patients by considering some of the insights into the human mind that psychology is able to give us.

EMOTIONS

Arriving at the site of an accident or where a person has been suddenly taken ill, the paramedic is likely to encounter much emotion, including his or her own. We can think of emotion as a mixture of feelings, behaviour and physiological changes. However, it is a striking feature of many emotions that the feelings and behaviour may be very different while the physiological changes that occur are similar (Lloyd and Mayes, 1984).

If we as paramedics can gain some understanding of where our emotions come from, we will be better equipped to deal with the distressed or angry patient. Schachter (Schacter and Singer, 1964) carried out the classic work in this field. He showed that emotion consists of two components: arousal which leads to widespread autonomic nervous system activity (such as increase in pulse and blood pressure); then we label our emotion according to cues that we take from the immediate situation we are in, and previous experience of similar situations. Emotion is therefore a combination of some arousing event and the cues we take from the immediate environment which determine how we will react.

Schachter's original work is now some 20 years old and considerable debate has surrounded his findings, but they are still widely accepted and form the basis for much work into understanding human emotion.

Significance of Schachter's Ideas

What then is the significance of these ideas for the paramedic out in the field? We may consider an accident or a sudden illness as an arousing event that will turn on the patient's emotional arousal, and the emotions and behaviour that follow will depend on the cues they receive from their environment. The paramedic and other persons in the vicinity will therefore play a major part in determining the emotional response displayed by the patient.

The Hostile and Aggressive Patient

The paramedic may be confronted with patients who are hostile and aggressive, or who are upset and crying. Whatever end of the emotional spectrum patients are on, they are less likely to be co-operative if they are emotionally disturbed, which is to their own detriment—and possibly the paramedic's if they are angry enough! A similar comment applies to family and friends, for if they are emotionally distressed or disturbed, vital information may be missed, a proper assessment of the patient may not be possible and extra stress is suffered by all concerned. It should also be remembered that the physiological changes associated with increased emotion may be very harmful for the patient.

Do not respond to provocation and become angry yourself as this will only give the patient yet more aggressive cues. This may well be easier said than done, but paramedics should try to learn to control their own feelings in such a situation and remain outwardly calm even though inwardly feeling very different. At all times the basic principle is to remember that the way you behave will give cues to the patient that will affect his or her emotional state.

The Patient with Myocardial Infarction

A particularly important example of this problem is patients who have just suffered an acute myocardial infarction or who are suffering from angina. The more distressed they become, the greater the activity of the sympathetic nervous system. One of the main effects of sympathetic stimulation is to increase heart rate and cardiac output, thereby increasing the work the heart has to do, so if it is damaged or its normal function is severely impaired, this is clearly to be avoided. Paramedics must therefore, by their own behaviour, give the patient calming and reassuring cues, rather than those that will provoke fear and anxiety; as a result they will lessen the workload on the damaged myocardium, improving the patient's prospects of survival every bit as much as by any technical wizardry.

The Wounded Patient

In the wounded patient, whether the wounds are a result of combat or even self-inflicted, heightened emotional behaviour may lead to further blood loss by increasing cardiac output as described above, in addition, if the patient refuses to be cooperative wound dressing may not be possible, while increased physical activity due to fear and agitation will also increase blood loss. The paramedic can do much to control bleeding and improve wound care without even laying a hand on the patient by simply giving calming, anxiety-reducing cues.

Sympathetic nervous system arousal as a result of heightened emotion may lead to marked changes in vital signs: blood pressure, respiratory rate and pulse may all be elevated. Emotional status must therefore be taken into account when interpreting such signs.

Modifying the Patient's Emotional State

Schachter's work suggests that we can modify the patient's emotional state to his benefit by the way we handle the situation and the cues we provide. Thus if we wish to minimise distress and anxiety we should try to remove such factors from the patient's immediate environment. The paramedic therefore needs a calm and confident manner whatever the situation. For example, if there is a distressed relative or agitated onlooker, it may be better for the patient if such a person is removed.

The paramedic must therefore not get caught up in the emotion of the situation. A calm approach followed by a rapid assessment is the essential start to your intervention, the aim being then to gain control of whatever is happening. Always be prepared and expect the unexpected.

Variance between Cultures

Emotion will also depend upon previous experience, a factor we can do little about. However, we also need to be aware that patients from different ethnic backgrounds or cultures may behave and display their emotions in very different ways. This difference should be accepted for what it is worth, an expression of the richness and diversity of the human race, not a behaviour that is to be condemned as 'soft' or 'unmanly'. It is not the paramedic's role to pass judgement on patients.

GRIEF AND BEREAVEMENT

On occasions our skills will be to no avail; the patient is already dead when the ambulance arrives or they die in the ambulance en route to hospital. In these situations, while nothing further may be done for the deceased, we should remember the family and friends, as much may be done for them by sympathetic and understanding care. It is important therefore to look at bereavement and grief to see how people may behave, especially in the initial period when emergency personnel are likely to be involved.

The Terminally Ill Patient

The majority of people in the western world die in old age and as a result of a long-term illness. Carr (1981) points out that most fatally ill people realise at some stage that they will not recover.

Yet despite the fact that at least 50% of such persons are aware that the outcome of their illness will be death, one study showed (Cartwright *et al.*, 1973) that only about 15% of terminally ill cancer patients, but 90% of their relatives had been told of their prognosis by a doctor.

In caring for terminally ill patients, emergency personnel need to be aware of this gap that appears to exist between what relatives have been told and what the patient knows. The resistance that still exists among some members of the medical profession to telling the patient their true prognosis calls for considerable tact and diplomacy at times.

Life-threatening Illness or Injury

Moving on from the terminally ill patient who has been living with death for some time, we must now look at sudden illness or injury which may be life-threatening—or which the patient may perceive in that way, which is just as important.

Kubler-Ross (1969) describes stages of denial, anger, bargaining, depression and acceptance among patients facing death in a terminal illness. But these may also be recognised in the critically injured patient if conscious. In a critical situation the paramedic should not be surprised to see the patient denying the seriousness of their condition, or displaying great anger, fear or anxiety.

A cool head is particularly important in this situation as the patient is in need of great support and understanding in what may well be their final minutes of consciousness. Most patients, however, lose consciousness before dying, so they are unaware of the moment of death. Saunders (1977) describes death as accompanied by a feeling of distance and sliding away, a point that is easy to forget in the hurly-burly of an attempted resuscitation. At all times the death of a patient should be accompanied by as much dignity as possible.

Bereavement, Family and Friends

We must now turn our attention to how family and friends will cope with the loss of a loved one, often in sudden and dramatic circumstances.

Hinton (1972) described grief as consisting of a series of stages, though they must not be thought of as a logical orderly sequence through which the person progresses. Human beings are too complex for that. Hinton described shock, denial, anxiety, depression, guilt and a wide variety of the physical signs of anxiety as the typical stages of the grieving process. They may be accompanied by searching behaviour, suicidal thoughts, idealisation of the lost person, panic, and a heightened incidence of physical and psychological disorders.

The grieving process occupies a lengthy period of time. Paramedics, however, will be more concerned with the immediate shock phase rather than the longer-term stages of despair and recovery. However, they should be aware that the relative of a dead patient is going to feel the effects of that death for a considerable period of time in many profound and highly significant ways.

How best then to tell relatives the worst news of all? Simply and directly is the best way. They will need the information in the simplest form in order to comprehend what they are being told. The initial response may vary from a daze of disbelief through total denial to stoical silence and apparent acceptance. All are grieving equally and feeling the loss just as severely, they are merely showing it in different ways.

Disbelief and Denial

The initial disbelief that commonly occurs may lead to the bereaved talking to the deceased as though alive or to displays of affection such as kissing or holding hands. The denial of death may be extreme and accompanied by great feelings of anger and guilt, a common reaction of which the paramedic must be aware. As the nearest target for displacement of such feelings, the paramedic may be on the receiving end of the bereaved person's despair and anger. Reacting will only make things worse; rather you should see the person's anger for what it is, a normal reaction to bereavement not a deliberate attack on your professional competence. Keep cool and let the person vent his or her feelings. The author vividly recalls seeing the father of a dead 8-year-old child picking the body off the resuscitation trolley in the accident unit and attempting to walk home carrying the body, convinced that the child was merely asleep. It took a great deal of tact and diplomacy to resolve that particular situation.

Alternatively, the paramedic should not be fooled by a person's stoical response; that reaction needs just as much support and understanding. On no account should the bereaved relative be left alone, and every effort should be made to find somebody to accompany him or her, a friend if possible or the next-door neighbour. If all else fails, serious consideration should be given to taking the relative to hospital, though preferably in another vehicle such as a police car, so that person will not be left to cope with the grief alone.

Those who have experienced the sudden death of a loved one, child or adult, have frequently written of the numbness involved, the feeling of utter despair, of being unable to think or act in any constructive, logical way. The paramedic needs to see this as a likely reaction of the bereaved, and be prepared to think for them in even the most basic matters until relatives or friends arrive who are slightly removed from the deceased and can assist in a more positive manner. Relatives often want to see and kiss their loved one before the body is removed, and they should be allowed this last wish. The possibility of stress-induced illness in relatives, such as heart attack or an acute asthmatic episode, should also be considered.

Cot Deaths

Perhaps one of the most difficult of all situations to be faced is the cot death. It is a mistake to think that parents grieve less for the loss of a baby than they do for the loss of a child—the pain is just as great, and is accompanied by massive feelings of guilt. The suffering of parents is made much worse when they are told little of what is happening and why. They suffer a cold and clinical reception at hospital, are given little information, and then are visited by the police who are obliged to investigate every cot death, thus compounding their suffering and despair. Paramedics can do little for the parents after the infant has reached hospital, but they can ensure that these mistakes are not made before the hospital system grinds its relentless way over such parents.

The Foundation for the Study of Infant Deaths has produced guidelines for hospital accident and emergency staff which, among other things, emphasise privacy, understanding, information and above all the chance to see and hold the dead infant. There is no reason why such principles should not apply in the prehospital situation; although the paramedic may be particularly disturbed by the suggestion that the parents should be allowed to see and hold their dead baby. Obviously if active resuscitation is underway, this will not be feasible, however in many cot death situations the infant is very obviously dead when the emergency services arrive. An attempt may be made on the way to hospital for the psychological wellbeing of the parents, who will then feel that everything possible was done for their infant, even though the paramedic knows full well it is a lost cause. Often, it is only by holding the dead infant in their arms that the parents can fully comprehend the fact of death. The necessary grieving process can then begin, and begin it must, for a failure to grieve fully for the death of a loved one may have severe long-term psychiatric complications.

The dilemma of whether to attempt resuscitation even though the situation is obviously hopeless is a real one. Are you unduly raising the parent's hopes, giving them the comfort that everything possible was done, or salving your own conscience? The answer lies with the individual paramedic in the real situation, not in the pages of this book. Ask yourself, if you were the child's parent, what would you prefer?

ACCIDENTS, EMERGENCIES AND CHILDREN

Emergency personnel will often find that their patient is a young child, or that children are present at the scene. Children need special attention as they see and understand the world differently from adults. The famous Swiss psychologist Jean Piaget has worked experiment and observation together into a very influential theory of how children develop which has considerable implications for emergency personnel.

Piaget's Theory of Child Development

In Piaget's theory (Mussen, 1979) we see children as continually trying to make sense of their world as they grow up. They progress from simply learning to grip things and then to walk, as infants, through various stages to be able to think in the adult way that we take for granted.

From Birth to Age 4

According to Piaget we should first look at the early months of life, up to an age of about 18 months. Here one of the first things that infants have to learn is that objects are permanent. To 6-month-old children, if an object cannot be seen then it no longer exists; that object could be the paramedic or anybody else, they have no idea of permanence. This idea usually develops by the time infants are 1 year old, a stage described as *egocentric* when they cannot see themselves as separate from the outside world.

Between the ages of 2 and 4, the children are in the stage of *preconceptual thought*: they still seem to see themselves as the most important people, the centre of what is happening. They have also discovered independence and seek to demonstrate this by refusing to do whatever they are asked.

It should be understood that when toddlers insist upon their wants being seen to immediately even though their mother may be injured or ill, they are not being selfish, merely exhibiting normal behaviour for their age.

Similarly toddlers who refuse to cooperate are demonstrating their independence rather than trying to be awkward, this being more an adult trait. We are all familiar with toddlers in the supermarket having a foot-stamping tantrum because they cannot get their own way. They cannot see that other members of the family have different wishes so they run away in protest to show their independence of action. These are typical behaviours in children of this age, and when confronted by a fractious 3-year-old patient or offspring of the patient, try to recall the supermarket example to understand why the child is behaving in this way. Firmness, kindness and understanding are required, together with a massive helping of patience.

From Ages 4 to 7

Between the ages of 4–7 years, Piaget considers children to be at a stage where they display *intuitive thought*. They begin to see things from other people's point of view, which starts making them more amenable to reason. But they still do not think like an adult—they cannot, for example, reverse a thought pattern. So although children of this age can now begin to see that there are more things to consider than their own point of view, their thought processes are very simple and naive compared to those of an adult.

From Ages 7 to 11

As children get older, between say 7 and 11 years of age, we are dealing with what is called the *concrete operational stage* of child development. Children are now capable of logical thought, but only in a very literal way. Everything is taken at its face value, so when we explain what is happening to children of this age we must do so in simple terms, remembering that they may well take everything said at face value.

Take an 8-year-old child with a leg injury that may well be a fracture. You want to immobilise the fracture in a splint and try to elevate the leg a little. You explain about the bones being broken, and the splint being needed to stop them rubbing together which will cause pain, and the child will probably understand, but go on to discuss tissue swelling causing pressure on nerve endings which in turn will cause pain, hence the need to elevate the leg, and you will lose your patient's understanding. Such abstract thought will be too difficult at this age to follow. *Caution*: remember that any joking comments about cutting off the leg may well be taken quite literally by the child, with awful results.

From Ages 12 to 14

It is in the age range 12–14 that children finally learn to think in the more abstract adult way. The ages that children reach these different stages of thought can vary considerably, and it is wise not to think of them as well-marked-out steps that will be rigidly adhered to; rather children ease their way into each stage, gradually, with some degree of overlap in thought process.

Reactions to the Environment

As the child's thinking changes with age, so too will his or her reactions to the environment. Consider how a child might react to a stranger. A paramedic is a stranger to the child, so what should we expect? Mussen (1979) describes how an infant aged between 6 and 15 months displays stranger anxiety, crying when confronted with a stranger, however friendly and kindly the latter tries to be. By the age of 18 months the infant has learned to handle the situation, leaving the room or running to mother.

Crying and anxiety diminish as the developing mental powers allow the child to cope with the situation. So the paramedic should not be too disconcerted by the year-old infant who promptly bursts into tears, nor the slightly older toddler who runs straight to mother, at the first sight of you. That is normal.

Children and Death

Children have different ideas about death at different stages of development. Carr (1981) considers that up to age 5, children neither know nor fear death, separation anxiety and fear of abandonment being uppermost in their mind. Between the ages of 6 and 10, as the thought processes develop, so do fears about pain and wounds. But it is not until the age of 10 and above that children really begin to understand death as the permanent cessation of life.

Keeping Child and Parent Together

As separation anxiety is the main fear in young children, every attempt should be made to keep child and parent together. Many young children are best moved to hospital sat on their parent's lap in the back of the ambulance, where they can be treated easily. They will allow their parent to hold a dressing or oxygen mask, where they might baulk at a paramedic doing so. This also helps many parents to feel involved in their child's care, and the fact they can see what exactly is happening eases their anxieties.

PERCEPTION:
HOW WE SEE THINGS

Assessment and interpersonal reactions are key components of the paramedic's role. Good care can only be given if there has been a good assessment of the patient. How the paramedic relates to the patient is therefore an integral part of emergency care, consequently perception, the way we see other people and the way they see us, is an area we should examine.

Errors in Patient Assessment

Mental Shortcuts

How then do we make sense of the continual bombardment of information that we encounter every day? One view sees perception of people and situations as being dependent upon previous experience. However, there is more to it than that, for we appear to build up a series of rules of association about what we experience that allow us rapidly to make sense of our encounters with the world at large. These rules create what are effectively mental pigeonholes into which we fit the mass of incoming data that bombards us every day. By having this readymade mental filing system we come to perceive and make sense of what is around us.

There is a snag, however, for these mental shortcuts lead us into creating stereotypes. We tend to think of people as being typical, we build up rules that tell us that any male with a very short haircut, boots, and scruffy jeans is a skinhead and therefore likely to be aggressive. We might also add that he is likely to be a football hooligan and belong to the National Front. In fact none of these latter statements might be true; he could simply be on leave from the army, and helping a friend with some building work, hence the scruffy jeans and boots.

If we are not careful, therefore, we can miss out or ignore the individuality of people by deciding that because they are dressed in a certain way, a whole host of assumptions immediately apply. The result is the paramedic reacting inappropriately due to faulty assessment of the patient.

For example, elderly people are sometimes deaf, and they may sometimes be confused. However, to assume that all elderly patients encountered for the first time are deaf and confused could be a serious error of judgement. They may have excellent hearing and be as mentally alert as you if not more so! They would certainly find being shouted at or patronised quite offensive. It is possible to make similar errors about all manner of social and ethnic groups within society. Nobody is typical, we are all individuals with the right to be treated as such, and paramedics must never lose sight of that fact if they are to make a proper assessment and give first rate care.

First Impressions

There are various other lessons that we can learn from the study of perception. The old cliché that first impressions count has been shown to be true in an interesting series of experiments (Luchins, 1957). Patients' opinions of the emergency personnel will be largely determined therefore by that vital first encounter, so you must try to secure their understanding and co-operation. An unguarded word or careless comment could create an impression that will take a lot of hard work to turn into something more favourable, meanwhile you have made your own job more difficult by creating an unfavourable perception of yourself with the patient.

Similarly, beware the trap of judging your patients purely by the first few seconds of your encounter. By reserving judgement and getting to know them a little, you may form a very different opinion of your patients and their problems. A friendly, helpful manner, even in the face of initial hostility, will usually create a more favourable first impression, and it is this first impression that will count.

The Hedonistic Principle

A further aspect of perception that should be considered is what Jones and de Charms (1964) called the hedonistic principle. By this they mean that if a person's actions interfere with our pleasure we are more likely to judge those actions in a worse light than would have been the case otherwise. For example, if you receive a call just before a meal break or when you are nearly at the end of a shift, something is clearly interfering with your pleasure, and if you are not aware of this hedonistic principle it would be very easy to assess that patient in a much more negative way than might otherwise be the case. After all, patients do not deliberately break their legs just because they know you are coming up to your meal break! A little mental discipline is needed to set aside the disappointment of having your food delayed so that you can carry on and assess the patient objectively.

Prejudgement

Interesting experiments by Walster (1966) showed that in judging someone to be guilty or of having done something wrong, we are more influenced by the outcome of what the person did rather than by the deed itself. It should be noted here that the paramedic's job is not to judge patients; they treat, others may judge. Consider the drunk driver who crashes his or her car: Walster's work indicates that if he or she had seriously injured a child, as a result our perception of that person would be very different from what it would be if the driver alone had been injured. The act was the same—drunk driving—but the outcome was different, so our assessment is different.

Abnormal Behaviour

One final source of error in patient assessment was described by Jones and Davis (1965). They demonstrated that the more abnormal a person's behaviour was, the more likely we are to attribute that abnormality to the person than the environment. The paramedic called to the scene of an accident where someone is behaving strangely is more likely to attribute that behaviour to some problem within the patient, rather than look for a simple explanation which may lie in the environment.

For example, you may encounter an agitated man running around with no clothes on. Before automatically assuming that he has a serious mental problem, consider also that he may be doing it to win a bet, his clothes may have been stolen, he may have just fallen in a river and his clothes are soaking wet, all are possible simple explanations stemming from outside the person, a reflection of the environment, rather than a mental problem coming from within.

Might not odd behaviour in the ambulance on the way to hospital be associated with the alien environment inside the ambulance? It might not be alien to you, but it will be to the average member of the public. This is particularly true if the patient is a little confused after, for example, a head injury or a stroke.

PSYCHOLOGICAL EFFECTS OF DISASTER

An overwhelming disaster, natural or manmade, will have profound effects on the survivors. Their behaviour will be significantly affected, and so will the work of the paramedic in dealing with them.

Initial Reactions

Miller (1974) describes the phenomenon frequently reported from disasters whereby survivors at first feel that they are the sole sufferer, the only person involved. Wolfenstein (1957) interprets this as being part of a feeling of abandonment related to childhood feelings of separation anxiety in the absence of the mother. As the child shows great love and affection upon the mother's return, so the disaster victim responds with similar feelings towards rescuers.

Emergency personnel at the scene of a disaster should not be surprised, therefore, if the initial response of a survivor is an apparent lack of concern for others involved. It is survivors' first response to think the disaster has only happened to them.

Many writers have described how survivors at first appear emotionless, unresponsive and generally very strained. Wolfenstein (1957) coined the phrase 'disaster syndrome' for this well-recognized state, suggesting that this inhibited emotional response helps people to deny the reality of what has happened, a self-defence mechanism. The horror of the event is so great that it cannot be understood or accepted at first, so it is initially denied while the person gradually comes to terms with what has happened. The intense fear associated with a disaster may only be fully experienced by the victims several days afterwards, so effective is this denial mechanism.

When arriving at the scene of a disaster, emergency personnel should not expect survivors to display great initiative. Apathy and disinterest are likely reactions, even to the point of further endangering their lives or at least not being very cooperative with rescue personnel. Here again, one must avoid judgemental attitudes: do not assume that uncooperative survivors are weak or selfish, they will simply be displaying a normal human response to an overwhelming catastrophe. It should also be noted that the most seriously injured casualties tend to be the least demanding due to their poor condition. An objective assessment is crucial; avoid becoming involved in the emotion of the situation.

The Post-disaster Situation

The anger found in grief may also be found in a post-disaster situation. As the numbness and apathy wear off, anger and guilt rise to the surface together with a great need to talk about what happened and those who died. If survivors show a need to talk, let them; it is an essential part of the recovery process after being involved in a disaster

In a major disaster, therefore the survivors will need a great deal of help and guidance as they have probably been rendered incapable of self-help by the psychological trauma of what has happened to them. Apparently uninjured survivors may still be casualties, but in a less obvious way.

Radiophobia

We have so far considered a situation in which those affected are readily identifiable. However, the late 20th century is the nuclear age, and as events at Chernobyl in the USSR have demonstrated, it is possible for people to become casualties even though they live many miles away from the scene of the disaster, and may be totally unaware that any untoward event has happened. The nuclear age has brought with it a new form of phobia—radiophobia. Radiation cannot be seen, heard, or felt, and it has no smell, so how do we know whether or not we have been explosed to it? The general public are rightly afraid of radiation.

The significance of this fear for emergency personnel is that if there were another major incident involving nuclear material, there would probably be panic and alarm. Large numbers of the population near Three Mile Island fled the scene as news spread of the stricken state of the reactor there. It is possible that a similar reaction would occur in the United Kingdom in a similar situation. In planning to deal with the consequences of a nuclear disaster, emergency personnel should take on board this radiophobia and the likely effect it may have on the general population, who may not behave in the rational way that we fondly imagine.

CONCLUSIONS

We may summarise this chapter by stating that there is much more to emergency care than dealing with obvious injuries and medical illness. An understanding of some basic psychology goes a long way in improving prehospital care. The paramedic will find it hard not to get caught up in the emotion of the situation. However, one must concentrate on the priorities of assessing and caring for the casualties in such a way that those who need care most urgently are the first to receive it. The numbing effect of disaster may lead to those most seriously injured making least fuss, which in turn raises the possibility that they may be missed in the initial chaos. The quiet victim is often more seriously injured than the more vociferous one, and also a person's physical injuries may make him or her incapable of calling for help.

Remember at all times that patients are also people with a whole complex range of mental activities occurring simultaneously as their more obvious physical functioning. Paying attention to what is happening inside your patient's head is just as important as what is happening elsewhere in the body, and is essential to ensure a high standard of hospital care.

References

Carr T. (1981) In Griffiths D. (ed.) *Psychology and Medicine*. London: Macmillan.

Cartwright A. *et al*. (1973) *Life Before Death*. London: Routledge.

Hinton J. M. (1972) *Dying*. London: Penguin.

Jones E., de Charms R., (1964) Changes in social perception as a function of personal relevance of behaviour. *Sociometry*, 75–85.

Jones E., Davis K. E. (1965) From acts to dispositions. In Berkowitz L. (ed.), *Advances in Experimental Social Psychology*, **2**: 219–266. New York: Academic Press.

Kubler-Ross E. (1969) *On Death and Dying*. London: Tavistock.

Lloyd P., Mayes A. *et al*. (1984) *Introduction to Psychology*. London: Fontana.

Luchins A. (1957) Primacy recency in impression formation. In Houland I. C. (ed.), *The Order of Presentation in Persuasion*. New Haven, Conn: Yale University Press.

Miller J. (1974) *Aberfan, A Disaster and its Aftermath*. London: Constable.

Mussen P. H. (1979) *Child Development and Personality*. New York: Harper and Row.

Saunders C. (1977) Dying they live. In Feifel H. (ed.), *New Meanings of Death*. New York: McGraw-Hill.

Schachter S., Singer, J. E. (1962) Cognitive social and physiological determinants of emotional state. *Psychological Review*, **69**: 379–399. Quoted in *Introduction to Psychology*, pp. 336–337. Hilgard E., Atkinson, R., Atkinson R. (1979) *Introduction to Psychology*. New York: Harcourt Brace Jovanovich.

Walsh M. (1985) *Accident and Emergency Nursing, A New Approach*. London: Heinemann.

Walster E. (1966) Assignment of responsibility for accidents. *Journal of Personal and Social Psychology*, 5:508–16.

Wolfenstein M. (1957) *Disaster*. Glencoe: The Free Press.

12. Mental Illness and Behavioural Problems

INTRODUCTION

Emergencies in mental health are perhaps less easy to deal with than physical ones. It is relatively easy to recognise a wound or fracture, but to try to fathom what is going on inside someone's head is much more difficult. There is a greater element of unpredictability, and therefore greater need for ingenuity and improvisation by the paramedic. The person who manifests disturbed behaviour requires tact and careful handling by the paramedic. However, it should be remembered that disturbed behaviour is not confined to the mentally ill; many other people in emergency situations behave in a disturbed way.

In the past the medical profession has tended to try to categorise people suffering from mental illness in the same way as physical illness—by giving disease titles to certain types of behaviour which then labels that behaviour as a discrete illness, different from other types of behaviour or illnesses. While there is great validity in this approach to physical disease, it has been called into question as the best way of dealing with mental illness. Writers such as Cooper (1980) consider (a) that human behaviour is too complex to be divided up in this way; and (b) this labelling of people is a means of exerting social control over people who are not ill, but just different from society's norm.

In this chapter a detailed description of different psychiatric conditions has therefore been avoided, and broader headings (which still reflect conventional psychiatric wisdom) have been used. The paramedic is more concerned with handling an emergency situation than with the finer points of psychiatric diagnosis, so consideration of behaviour in broad terms is therefore justified. Experience of the reality of emergency situations on the street, or in someone's home supports this broad approach.

THE PSYCHOTIC PATIENT

Hilgard, Atkinson and Atkinson (1987) consider that a psychotic illness involves a serious disorder of thought and behaviour, and frequently loss of contact with reality. Sufferers, therefore, have little or no insight into their illness; in fact, they may not see themselves as ill at all. Help and treatment therefore become much more difficult, and patients may interpret the actions of emergency personnel in a very different light from which they are intended.

Psychotic patients may withdraw from reality and live in their own fantasy world, failing to respond to what is happening around them, or display inappropriate emotions that do not fit their situation. Disturbance of thought processes lead to hallucinations that may consist of hearing voices or involve the other senses. Delusional ideas may develop, often paranoid, or they may represent ideas of grandeur out of all keeping with reality.

Schizophrenia

This diagnostic label applies to a group of mental disorders characterised by a disintegration of the thought processes. Sheahan (1973) describes how this gradual disintegration of rational thought leads to disordered emotion and conduct coupled with increasing withdrawal from the person's environment.

It is the disordered thought process that will often reveal itself to the paramedic as the first indication of schizophrenia: the conversation will wander in an inconclusive and sometimes bizarre fashion; simple questions may produce vague and woolly answers; schizophrenia sufferers' thinking is disjointed and illogical, they may stop in mid-sentence and totally change the thread of their conversation. I remember asking one lady the time and being told it was half past Wednesday! It is as if their train of thought has run into a brick wall, hence the description of this phenomenon as *thought block*.

The person's perception may be disturbed by hallucinations which commonly consist of hearing voices, so-called *auditory* hallucinations. The other senses can be affected in a similar way. It has to be emphasised that to these patients, the hallucination is very real, they really do hear that voice as a real voice, sometimes giving a running commentary on what is happening around them or telling them what to do next.

Emotionally, schizophrenia sufferers may become very flat, showing a lack of feeling and talking in a dull monotone. They may also show a disharmony between what they say and the way it is said known as *inappropriate effect*; thus sad statements, for example, may be made with a happy voice.

Emergency personnel will tend to be involved with the person suffering from a schizophrenic type of illness during an acute flare-up. Very disturbed and bizarre behaviour is possible in these situations due to the disturbed thought processes and perceptions of reality that the person is experiencing. He or she is very unlikely to have much insight into these problems during the acute episodes.

The reality of patients' voices may lead them to perform some very strange actions. Unfortunately, if paranoid ideas creep into these voices, there is a potential for violence against others or themselves. Sirhan Sirhan, Robert F. Kennedy's assassin is described by Hilgard, Atkinson and Atkinson (1987) as suffering from a schizophrenic illness with paranoid delusions.

Recognising the Problem

If called to situations where people who appear to be suffering from strange or disordered thought processes are exhibiting strange behaviour paramedics should ask themselves to what extent these persons are in touch with reality. If the answer is that they do not seem to be; they appear to be talking to voices that the paramedics cannot hear; or perhaps they are talking of picking up messages from the TV or radio; if their thoughts are jumbled and it is difficult to follow any coherent, logical conversation, then a schizophrenic type of illness is a likely explanation.

Emergency personnel must beware the trap of labelling anybody behaving strangely (strangely to you, that is) as psychotic or schizophrenic. These are labels with very adhesive qualities, easy to apply and very difficult to remove! Look for alternative explanations for the behaviour, such as drug abuse or some medical condition, before settling on a psychotic type episode as the explanation.

Management of the Psychotic Patient

When confronted with this type of situation it is important first of all to try to identify yourself very clearly both with your name, and as a person who is there to try to help. The patient's interpretation of who you are and what you are trying to do may be very different from yours.

The similarity between the traditional ambulance crew uniform and police uniform may lead people to believe they are being arrested by the police; any paranoid delusions may be considerably heightened by such a belief. Unexplained actions and comments made out of the hearing of a person suffering from paranoid ideas may take on extremely powerful meanings which could be very disturbing. We therefore need to explain carefully and clearly to the patient all actions that are taken, so that the risk of misunderstanding is minimised; try to avoid the temptation to make quiet asides to other colleagues within sight of the patient. It cannot be emphasised enough that the person's perception of reality may be *very* disturbed with the result that even the most innocent action or comment could assume great or threatening significance.

If patients are hallucinating or expressing delusional thoughts, they should not be confronted or denied outright. Argument will only tend to make the problems worse, as these ideas and hallucinations are very real to the patient.

For example, how would you feel if two men dressed a little like police officers suddenly came into your room and denied you were reading this book, told you it does not exist and is all a figment of your imagination? If they persisted in their arguments, and then told you that they would have to take you away against your wishes and lock you up if you continue to believe that this book exists, and also persist in the delusion that they are ambulancemen (or women), you would be angry and possibly struggle and become violent if they laid hands on you. So it is for psychotic patients—to them their hallucinations and delusions may be just as real.

The best approach is to indicate that you understand what they are experiencing, that they are hearing voices or that you know they think the CIA and MI5 have a contract out on their life. However, you should also indicate that you cannot hear the voice yourself, or that you have no knowledge of any contracts on their life but you would like to help because they seem to be having problems. You therefore avoid colluding with the delusions or hallucinations, but at the same time manage to avoid confrontation by denying their existence.

It is helpful if the patients can be located in a quiet area. Try to remove stimulating factors such as noise, lots of activity, or any particular person whose presence seems to cause agitation. They should be allowed to talk freely; let them ventilate their feelings while you sit and listen. Pay attention, sit slightly forward, engage in eye contact, adopt an open posture with arms and legs unfolded, make a few helpful vocal gestures such as comments like 'I see', 'yes', 'carry on' that show you are interested in what the person has to say. This approach often has a calming effect; you can begin to build a relationship, as patients start to feel they can trust you, and the whole situation is defused.

Time spent in this way can be very productive. Patients' behaviour can be controlled without the need for force, always the very last resort. The paramedic can gain a lot of information about the patients, and begin to assess just how much they are in touch with reality. The other member of the crew can meanwhile be having a discreet conversation with members of the family, friends or others in the vicinity to find out as much background information as possible. They may also be in touch with the person's general practitioner or the local hospital accident and emergency unit. Given the long-term nature of schizophrenia, it is likely that the family will be able to confirm your suspicions, or the general practitioner will be aware of the picture and can start to make appropriate arrangements with medical colleagues. The person may not yet have been diagnosed as suffering from a schizophrenic type of illness (the age of onset is typically early adulthood, 18–25 years), so this line of action may not be as simple as it sounds.

Patients may not, of course, be as cooperative as we have indicated so far. It is very tempting to try to trick them into the ambulance to take them to hospital, when otherwise they would not willingly agree to go. However, the likely outcome when they realise they have been tricked, will only be a major outburst on arrival, or worse still, while still on the road. In addition, all trust will have been destroyed, paranoid patients' worse fears will have been confirmed, and the work of the hospital staff in helping them get over their acute illness will have been made that much harder.

The use of force to remove a person to hospital is very much the last resort: it will destroy any trust that there might have been between patient and those trying to help; once restraint is released the patient is likely to be very angry and the patient–caring staff relationship may be seriously compromised.

Every attempt should therefore be made to obtain the patient's cooperation in going to hospital voluntarily. The usefulness of other family members should not be underestimated in this situation. While an acutely psychotic patient can be one of the most difficult with whom emergency personnel have to deal, it is worth remembering that the same person in another time and place might be regarded as a great holy man or prophet by his ability to see visions and hear the voices of God.

Depression

At times we all have felt sad and low; we have all felt depressed. However, these moods are as nothing compared to an anguish and despair so black that the only logical solution is to end life itself. This is the despair of depression that has become so intense as to constitute a life-threatening condition.

Depression of this severity is characterised by an unrelenting mood of despair. Sufferers feel both helpless and hopeless, guilty and unworthy. Withdrawal into a world of black desolation leaves them unable to communicate with the outside world, and anyway, what is the point? Physical changes accompany the depression, there is loss of weight and appetite, difficulty in sleeping, early morning waking. All who have worked night duty will be familiar with the dead hour of 4 am when even the most cheerful person feels down; how much worse it is then for the depressed person waking at this hour. Impotence or amenorrhoea (lack of menstruation) may accompany the condition.

People suffering from this degree of depression have a life-threatening illness. They may well decide that the only way to solve their problems is to commit suicide, and may discuss the idea quite openly. Talk of suicide, however veiled the hint may appear, should be taken seriously.

The paramedic may be confronted by withdrawn, uncommunicative individuals. Help has often been summoned by another person, as depressed people may be unable to ask for help themselves. Occasionally they may be found on the edge of suicide—literally, if there is a well-known jumping location such as the Clifton suspension bridge in Bristol. Fortunately such dramatic encounters are rare, but they can happen.

Management of the Depressive Patient

The person needs to be approached sympathically rather than with a brusque 'pull yourself together' manner. Start by sitting down, identifying yourself as a person who wants to help, and try to talk to the person. Conversation may be very difficult due to the person's extreme withdrawal, but emergency personnel should see this as a sign of illness. In view of the high suicide risk in this group it is as well if the depressive patient is not left alone, and every effort should be made to give medical help as soon as possible. Use should be made of family and friends as appropriate.

As depressed patients are likely to be fairly uncommunicative it is all the more important that they believe that anything they do say will be listened to. You must therefore be a sympathetic and patient listener. Due to the passivity found in depression it will probably be easier to transfer such people to hospital than someone in an acutely psychotic, disturbed state. *Caution*: always remember the suicide risk.

Manic States

Manic conditions are characterised by overactivity and excitement (Hilgard, Atkinson and Atkinson, 1987). Such people will be continually active, they cannot sit still, they pace up and down, speech becomes rapid and loud. Attempts to interfere with what they are doing can provoke aggression. Behaviour is extremely impulsive with the patients likely to do anything as soon as the idea enters their head, this includes sexual impulses. Delusions of power and grandeur may also be present.

If called to people showing such wild and excitable behaviour, emergency personnel should also consider the possibility of drug abuse (LSD or amphetamines are most likely) or of an acute schizophrenic episode. It is important again to establish how much contact with reality patients have in order to assess the chances

of this being an acute psychotic episode as opposed to just somebody being very excited. Try to assess their thought patterns: are
they logical? Is there evidence of hallucinations or delusions?

Management of Manic Conditions

Our approach needs to be similar to those discussed above. Identify yourself, point out that you are a helper, be prepared to
listen, and try to calm matters down by your own manner as
much as by any other means. Tactful enquiry needs to be made
about the possibility of drug use or whether the person has had
similar episodes in the past. Allow for impulsive behaviour, it is
part of the illness; attempts to thwart this may well lead to outbursts of aggression.

Urgent transfer to hospital is needed for patients in a manic
state as they may come to great harm or harm others. This may
be possible with persuasion, and certainly again every effort
should be made to get them there voluntarily. Remember to use
family and friends if possible to persuade the patient to cooperate. A struggling, handcuffed patient sandwiched between
two policemen with a paramedic sitting on top of them is the last
thing the local accident and emergency department or psychiatric admissions unit will want. The Mental Health Act (pp.
178–80) may need to be resorted to, if persuasion fails.

Manic Depression

Some unfortunate people suffer from both manic and depressive
episodes; this is known as manic depression. We all have mood
swings, some days are great when we feel on top of the world, and
others are awful when nothing goes right and we end up feeling
really miserable. But for some people the extremes of these
normal mood swings are much greater, and they will experience
episodes of profound depression lasting weeks before returning
to a fairly stable 'normal' level of functioning. Months later, however, they may become manic in their excitement and again need
hospitalisation. During the intervening stable periods they often
have great insight into the nature of their illness.

We may summarise this consideration of psychotic conditions by
reminding the paramedic that you need not be too concerned
with the details of psychiatric diagnosis. The key factors to con-

sider are patients' behaviour and thought; and are they in touch with reality? Is there evidence of hallucinations or delusions? What previous mental history is there? Always expect the unexpected, be prepared to listen in a calm manner and clearly identify yourself as a helper. And finally remember that these are emergencies in just the same way as a heart attack or a diabetic coma, and can have equally fatal outcomes if not handled correctly.

ANXIETY AND NEUROSES

We are all familiar with anxiety; it is an essential tool for survival. Without anxiety, for example, we would not wait for the traffic lights to turn green before driving on, nor would we look carefully before walking across the road. Yet in some people it can get out of hand, and become a crippling illness with acute episodes needing the intervention of the emergency services. This neurotic anxiety is described by Ryecroft (1978) as anxiety provoked by a situation which should give no grounds for it. Such anxiety may seem absurd and ridiculous to others, and even to the person suffering from it. There is, then, an element of insight that is lacking in a psychotic condition.

It is the failure to master and control anxiety that leads to a neurotic condition. Fears may be focused on a particular type of object or situation, for example, spiders; or open spaces (agoraphobia), or be of a more free-floating, non-specific type that leads to general anxiety quite capable of crippling the person's ability to live a normal life. The paramedic should note the physical effects that anxiety can have on the body. By stimulating the sympathetic nervous system, blood pressure, respiratory and pulse rates can all be raised quite substantially, an important fact to note when assessing the patient, as the paramedic may be led to try to explain such observations in terms of physical causes.

Anxiety

Anxiety states can lead to panic attacks and calls for emergency assistance. The picture that tends to greet emergency personnel is of a greatly distressed patient with a noticeably rapid respiratory rate and pulse. This rapid breathing (hyperventilation) can have serious effects: as the person is breathing out more carbon dioxide than normal, there is a disturbance of blood chemistry that leads to the condition known as tetany (not to be confused with tetanus). In this situation patients feel severe cramps and spasms of the abdominal muscles, and also have a characteristic spasm of the fingers known as carpopedal spasm (Fig. 12.1). These painful cramps can make people even more distressed and cause more hyperventilation setting up a vicious circle.

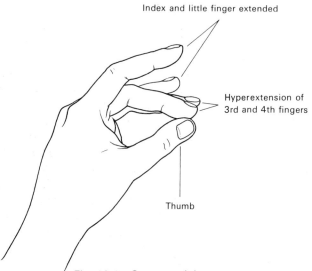

Index and little finger extended

Hyperextension of 3rd and 4th fingers

Thumb

Fig. 12.1   Carpo-pedal spasm

When dealing with people who appear to be greatly distressed in this way, try to calm everything down and carry out a quick assessment of the situation. Are they in touch with reality? If so, is there any obvious physical cause for their distress, such as an injury? If there is no obvious medical cause for the distress patients are feeling, then anxiety or some emotional upset should be considered. A calm reassuring manner and a willingness to listen will go a long way towards controlling the situation. Try to remove any obvious upsetting stimuli such as noise, or any individual who appears to be distressing the patient.

If patients are hyperventilating with painful spasms then the carbon dioxide levels must be restored to normal to relieve the spasm. This is done by getting patients to rebreathe the air they have just exhaled either simply with a paper bag or using a bag and mouthpiece from your resuscitation equipment. Explain to the patients what you are doing and why. The reaction to being asked to breathe into a brown paper bag is not likely to be instant cooperation unless an explanation is provided. In addition the paramedic will need to calm and reassure patients that all is well and ask them to concentrate on their breathing, making sure they breathe slowly.

Hysteria

Another aspect of neurosis that may be encountered is that of hysteria. Ryecroft (1978) describes how patients complain of physical symptoms without a physical cause; in other words no disease is present. The description is said to correspond to the patients' ideas of how their bodies work rather than the actual facts of anatomy and physiology: for example, they may insist that their legs are paralysed or that they have gone blind. It is worth noting that the person is not deliberately malingering, but really does feel the symptoms of which they are complaining.

If you are dealing with distressed patients and you suspect that their symptoms may be hysterical because you can find no obvious cause for them, you should still treat their complaints as real. There are two good reasons for doing so: (a) it is real to the patient, so saying 'There is nothing wrong with you, stop making such a fuss' will only anger the patient and family; (b) there is always the possibility that something may really be wrong, although it is not immediately obvious.

Caution: Here again, do not become judgemental about patients. Beware the trap of thinking 'Just another typical hysterical female'. People are individuals, not types. Further, plenty of males as well as females suffer from hysterical episodes.

PERSONALITY DISORDER

This is a very broad term applied to a wide range of problem behaviours. Sufferers of personality disorders are not mentally ill in that they are in touch with reality and quite aware of the consequences of their actions. The problem is that they do not seem to care about them. They do what they want, often at society's expense, with little or no regard for any suffering their actions may cause. One label applied to personalities in this group is psychopath, and such persons regularly come to the attention of emergency personnel, often causing considerable problems of management.

Psychopathy

Hilgard, Atkinson and Atkinson (1987) consider psychopaths as people lacking in any feelings of guilt or remorse for their actions, or regard for others. They will seek out what they want immediately, often acting on impulse. Other characteristics include a facility for lying, a constant need for thrills and a disregard for danger.

Given this description, it is not surprising that people with a psychopathic personality are seldom far from trouble, and may well suffer serious injury as a result of either accidents or violence. Walsh (1985) has described their potential for trouble in the accident and emergency department, especially if they have been drinking or using drugs. In addition to overt aggression and violence, lying, manipulation and threats are all possible, as is attention-seeking behaviour such as self-inflicting wounds or swallowing sharp objects. This may also be encountered outside the hospital.

Management of Psychopathy

The key point to remember when trying to handle this sort of behaviour is that, unlike the psychotic patient, these people know *exactly* what they are doing and are therefore responsible for their actions. We therefore recommend that no attempt be made to intervene physically if such patients are indulging in self-harm. These patients have a high potential for violence and you will only be rewarding the attention-seeking behaviour by giving them the attention they seek, especially if a crowd of onlookers is present as is often the case. Rewarding any sort of behaviour tends to lead to its repetition (Hilgard, Atkinson and Atkinson, 1987) so attempting a dramatic intervention only stores up trouble for the future.

It is best at the outset to set firm limits to acceptable behaviour. If psychopathic patients are prepared to stay within limits and cooperate, offer help and assistance, but if they are going to be disruptive, leave them to get on with it. Remember, psychopaths are *not* mentally ill, they fully understand what they are doing. If they wish to stand in the middle of the street and cut their arm with broken glass, *let them*. Attempts at forceful intervention may well be dangerous for the paramedic. Talk, keep cool, offer help if they want it, for now or later.

A firm approach is required, setting limits and treating psychopaths as responsible adults, but *do not* try to use force or coercion and beware being manipulated. 'If you don't do...then I'll...' is a frequently heard piece of manipulation or blackmail; emergency personnel cannot work under blackmail from patients. It is difficult apparently to refuse to try to help people in the street, but you cannot force somebody to accept treatment when they are refusing to cooperate. If necessary the police should be summoned to deal with the incident.

It is worth remembering that few psychiatrists will accept psychopaths into hospital for treatment as they do not consider they are mentally ill or that their behaviour will improve as a result of any treatment that may be offered in a hospital setting. They are also reluctant to invoke the Mental Health Act to deal with a psychopathic personality.

MUNCHAUSEN'S SYNDROME

This bizarre illness may well present itself to the emergency services without them even being aware of it. Walsh (1985) describes the patient as a person who gains frequent admissions to hospital, often in very dramatic emergency circumstances, with a story that turns out to be false. There is no significant physical illness, although the symptoms are accurately described by the patient, and signs such as coughing up blood or passing it in the urine will be well faked by careful deliberate self-injury (for example, making a small cut in the tongue or finger, and then squeezing a few drops of blood into the urine specimen).

The principal illnesses that are acted out are collapse and chest pain, abdominal pain, bleeding from various orifices, fits and psychiatric disturbance. Such persons tend to travel around the country obtaining hospital treatment by fraud, often at great

Table 12.1 Summary of Mental Health Act (1983). Adapted from MIND (1983)

Legislation	Criteria	Application	Medical recommendations	Effect
Section 4: Admission for assessment in an emergency	Admission for assessment required as a matter of urgent necessity	Nearest relative or approved social worker (ASW) Patient must be seen by applicant during the 24 hours before application is made	One written recommendation by any doctor, but if possible, one with previous knowledge of the patient	Patient detained for a maximum of 72 hours unless second medical opinion given and received by hospital management in that period. Provisions of Part IV on consent to treatment do not apply.
Section 136: Mentally disordered persons in public places	If a police constable finds a person in a public place who appears to be suffering from a mental disorder and is in immediate need of care or control	A police officer	Nil	Person can be taken to place of safety to be interviewed by ASW or doctor, such as accident and emergency department or police station. Maximum detention 72 hours
Section 135: Warrant to search for and remove patient	There is reasonable cause to suspect that a person believed to be suffering from a	ASW to a JP (on oath)	Nil	Police constable, ASW and doctor can enter patient's premises and remove him or her to a place of

	mental disorder has been ill-treated or neglected, or is unable to care for him or herself and lives alone			safety. Maximum detention 72 hours
Section 2: Admission for assessment	Mental disorder warranting detention in hospital for assessment and treatment; the patient ought to be detained in interests of own health and safety or for the protection of others	Nearest relative and ASW who must interview patient	Two doctors, one of whom must be approved under Section 12. Doctors not to be from same hospital	Patient detained for maximum of 28 days. Part IV applies for treatment without consent
Section 3: Admission for treatment	Mental illness or severe impairment, psychopathic disorder or mental impairment of a nature or degree which makes medical treatment in hospital appropriate	As for Section 2, but ASW cannot make an application if the nearest relative objects	As for Section 2	Patient detained for maximum of 6 months, renewable for a further 6, then for 1 year at a time

expense to the NHS. From my own experience in Bristol, I would estimate that one such person appears every two or three weeks, going the rounds. The problem is therefore quite serious, but as a paramedic you are in a most difficult situation, as initially you have to respond to the patient as a genuine emergency.

The reader may be interested to note the career of one such case traced by one of the authors, over a 31-day period before presentation at the accident and emergency department in Bristol in 1981. This young man of 25 had spent 26 of the previous 31 days in eight different hospitals in South Wales, Gloucestershire and Avon, with a variety of complaints ranging from having a head injury to an injured knee. You may work out for yourself the amount of time and money he cost the NHS!

THE MENTAL HEALTH ACT

The 1983 Mental Health Act allows for certain situations where, due to the lack of insight found in psychotic conditions, patients' wishes may be contrary to their best interests. Treatment, sedation and detention in a place of safety may therefore be carried out *against* the patient's wishes.

We have already emphasised the need for persuasion rather than force. However, there may be situations when persuasion fails, and due to the person's disturbed mental condition detention and treatment or observation are required. The Mental Health Act may then be used, but only with great caution, as it does represent a major breach of civil liberty and all staff must be careful to stay within the limits of the law as a result.

The key sections of the act most likely to affect paramedics are outlined in Table 12.1. When transferring mentally ill patients, always ascertain whether they are voluntary or detained under the Mental Health Act, and before setting out on the road obtain clarification concerning escorts, if this is an interhospital transfer rather than an emergency admission from home.

CONCLUSION:
GUIDELINES FOR MANAGING
MENTALLY ILL PATIENTS

In this section we attempt to translate into practice much of the theory discussed above in this chapter. The following are guidelines that ambulance crew should find helpful.

(1) You have no legal right to force people into an ambulance or to keep them there unless they are detained under a section of the Mental Health Act.

(2) Check that all relevant documents are in order if you are moving patients against their will under a Section of the Mental Health Act, otherwise you will be committing assault.

(3) If you are dealing with unsectioned patients who are unwilling to go to hospital, rely on persuasion, stressing the benefits of going to hospital, and trying to motivate them.

(4) If your powers of persuasion fail, avoid becoming involved in the situation as your vehicle and skills may be needed elsewhere. Explain the situation to control and request the presence of a doctor who can begin the sectioning procedure.

(5) Approach patients with caution: they may be carrying a weapon in their hand or on their person, which they may use suddenly and unexpectedly.

(6) The kitchen is the most likely source of weapons, so try to keep your patient away from there if possible.

(7) Beware rooms that lock on the inside such as the bathroom or toilet; patients may well lock themselves in such rooms and administer considerable self-harm while you are trying to get them out again.

(8) Always be aware of the possibility of a sudden change in mood or behaviour. Mentally ill persons may be illogical and quite unpredictable.

(9) If you are experiencing difficulties in transit and the patient is struggling, radio ahead to the accident and emergency department so they know what to expect, but choose your words carefully as the patient will probably

hear you. There is no point in pouring petrol on the flames! (Remove their shoes prior to loading if there is a possibility of violence.)

(10) Whilst in the ambulance ensure (for safety reasons) that a seat belt, or safety belt, if a stretcher patient, is always fastened around them.

(11) Should the patient be female, male ambulance crew are strongly advised to get a friend to accompany the patient in the back of the ambulance; there is always the risk of allegations of indecency.

(12) Make sure that the accident and emergency staff receiving the patient have *all* the relevant information.

(13) Remember that the police have the power both of arrest and to detain somebody under a section of the Mental Health Act if necessary. If you find people behaving in a disturbed fashion, but refusing to cooperate—for example, standing in the middle of the street cutting their wrists but refusing to go to hospital with you—then the best course of action is to call for police assistance. You would be unwise to tackle them yourself, but it would not create a good image of the ambulance service if you simply drove away.

References

Cooper D. (1980) *The Language of Madness*. Harmondsworth: Pelican.

Hilgard E., Atkinson R., Atkinson R. (1987) *Introduction to Psychology*, 2nd edn. New York: Harcourt, Brace and Jovanovich.

Mitchell, R. (1975) *Depression*. Harmonsworth: Penguin.

MIND (1983) *A Practical Guide to Mental Health Law*. London: MIND.

Ryecroft C. (1978) *Anxiety and Neurosis*. Harmondsworth: Penguin.

Sheahan J. (1973) *Essential Psychiatry*. Lancaster: MTP Press.

Walsh M. H. (1985) *Accident and Emergency Nursing, A New Approach*. London: Heinemann.

13. Suicide and Deliberate Self-harm

INTRODUCTION

Suicide, the deliberate taking of one's own life, runs at around 4000 cases per year in the UK, the majority of whom are male. Peak rates for this century were recorded in the 1930s and again in the late 1960s when the annual number was around the 5500 mark (Farmer and Hirsch, 1980). More recent figures show a slight increase. Self-poisoning is by far the commonest method used, followed by hanging and drowning.

The phrase 'deliberate self-harm' was proposed by Morgan (1979) to describe another phenomenon with which emergency personnel will quickly become familiar. Morgan was describing a large group of patients who either take an overdose of drugs or inflict wounds on themselves, often repeatedly but with no suicidal intent. It is not appropriate to describe them as attempting suicide; using the word overdose to describe such patients omits large numbers of persons who have self-inflicted injuries. These people clearly have related problems, and often the same person will indulge in both forms of behaviour.

To gain some idea of the scale of the problem, the numbers have grown from 23 900 admissions in 1961 from overdose, to 106 700 by 1977 (Walsh, 1985). Various other studies consistently place the number of cases attending hospital at substantially over 100 000 per year, although the spectacular rate of growth in the 1960s and 1970s has slowed down markedly. Table 13.1 shows that drug overdose is primarily a problem of the younger age groups, affecting women more than men, with over 60% of cases aged under 34.

Table 13.1   Distribution of Overdose by Age
From Hospital Inpatient Enquiry (1977)

Age group	Per cent	Ratio female:male
15–19	16.6	3.26
20–24	18.0	1.85
25–34	27.3	1.54
35–44	17.0	1.75
45–64	15.2	1.67
65–74	3.7	2.00
75+	2.0	1.15

Another aspect of the problem is that it mostly affects urban
areas: the poorest inner city parts and large council estates
known to have a high social problem profile (Walsh, 1982). The
multiple problems faced by people living in these areas, and the
lack of individual resources to deal with them, help to explain
deliberate self-harm as a means of problem-solving.

REASONS FOR
DELIBERATE SELF-HARM

A commonly encountered situation involves people who feel that
their spouse/girlfriend/boyfriend does not pay enough attention
to them, or is leaving. In an emotional scene an overdose of
tablets is taken, then after a suitable period of time the person
rings 999 or arranges for the overdose to be discovered in time.
This, of course, is where you enter the scene.

The aim of the person who has taken the overdose is to attract
attention or to make the spouse/girlfriend/boyfriend feel guilty,
'Look what you've made me do, it's all your fault', with the aim of
making the departing spouse/friend return, or to hurt them, or at
least to be noticed. However, suicide is *not* the aim.

Not all cases of self-poisoning are as simple as this, and emergency personnel will encounter some that are clearly suicidal.
However, the overwhelming majority of the 100 000 plus cases
seen every year fit into the above framwork. It is worth asking
yourself how the patients were discovered. If they tried to con-

ceal their overdose and escape discovery, then the attempt was likely to be a potential suicide; but if they immediately told somebody what they had done or dialled 999 themselves, this is much less likely to be a suicide attempt. Also if patients have only taken a small quantity of drugs, especially if these are drugs taken regularly, this again is unlikely to be a suicide attempt.

Caution: It is unwise to become overconfident in dealing with an apparently trivial overdose. Barraclough *et al.* (1974) made a detailed study of 100 successful suicides and found that 90% had received some sort of medical help within the year preceding their suicide, and 48% within the week. The idea of the suicide 'out of the blue' therefore does not hold up to examination, and when called to a person whose overdose has been reported, every effort should be made to persuade that person to go to the accident and emergency department with you.

HIGH-RISK FACTORS IN SUICIDE

The following is a checklist of high-risk factors that point to subsequent suicide, found by Tuckman and Youngman (1968) in a detailed follow-up of 3800 attempters:

(1) Age 45 or over
(2) Male
(3) Unemployed or retired
(4) Separated, divorced or widowed
(5) Living alone
(6) Poor physical health
(7) Having received medical treatment within the last 6 months
(8) Psychiatric disorder or alcoholism
(9) Use of self-directed violence rather than overdose
(10) Presence of a suicide note
(11) History of previous attempts.

The more factors present, the greater the suicidal intent is likely to be. Persons who had ten factors present were found to have almost ten times the subsequent suicide rate of those with only two to five factors. When summoned to a person who is reluctant to go with you to hospital, consider these factors outlined above; the more there are the greater the suicide risk involved and, consequently, the greater the need for medical help. As an alternative try to get the person's general practitioner to come to the home rather than taking the person to hospital.

We can summarise overdose behaviour by describing it as being most common amongst the younger age group, females more than males, and associated with deprived, poorer areas of towns. It is rarely suicidal in intent, being usually an impulsive act in response to some life crisis such as the break-up of a relationship.

It must be emphasised that the person may have taken a potentially fatal overdose without realising it. Tablets taken range from very powerful drugs prescribed by doctors through to ordinary mild painkillers bought over the counter in the chemists; many of these can be fatal, including the simplest of pain-relieving drugs such as paracetamol (Table 13.2) So every effort should be made to get the patient to hospital. If they refuse the general practitioner *must* be called to the home.

From the patient's point of view, there has been a major life crisis for which they need help. Failure to take them to a medical facility may have unpredictable and serious, possibly fatal effects. In hospital, the immediate medical problems posed by the drugs or wounds can be dealt with, and an expert psychiatric opinion obtained if necessary.

The problem remains of the person who refuses absolutely to go with you, even after attempts at persuasion by yourself, family and friends have failed. Patients have the right to refuse treatment unless they are detained under a specific section of the Mental Health Act (see Chapter 12), therefore you cannot force them to go to hospital. It is best to summon help from a general practitioner (preferably the patient's own) who can visit the scene, assess the patient, and if necessary begin the procedures required for compulsory detention and treatment under the Mental Health Act.

However, if the patient refuses to accompany you to the accident and emergency department, and even refuses to see a general practitioner, there is little else that can be done except to leave the patient and family with the assurance that should the patient have a change of mind, treatment will still be available.

Table 13.2 Drugs commonly Taken in Overdose

Salicylic acid (aspirin)
Effects
Increased respiratory rate, rapid pulse, tinnitus (ringing in the ears), nausea, vomiting and abdominal pain. Potentially fatal due to severe disturbances in metabolism. May be washed out up to 12 h after ingestion. Expert hospital treatment may be required depending on blood salicylate levels

Paracetamol (Panadol, Hedex, etc)
Effects
Severe liver damage may be caused by as little as 20 tablets, liver failure develops after 5–6 days. Potentially fatal if more than 20 tablets taken

Benzodiazepines (Valium, Mogadon, Librium, etc)
Effects
Drowsiness, ventilatory depression. Not fatal on their own, but the airway is greatly at risk due to coma and breathing will be very depressed

Tricyclic antidepressants (amitriptyline, imipramine, etc)
Effects
Cardiac arrhythmias, ventilatory depression, convulsions and coma. A potentially fatal overdose, though patients may be washed out up to 12 h after taking tablets. Cardiac monitoring on CCU is required.

Distalgesic
Effects
As for paracetamol, but also includes dextropropoxyphene, a mild narcotic which therefore causes a risk of respiratory depression

Barbiturates (Tuinal, Seconal, Sodium Amytal, etc)
Effects
Severe respiratory depression and arrest, hypothermia, coma. High potential for fatality

MANAGEMENT OF OVERDOSE

As with other conditions the first concern is with the basic ABC of resuscitation. If a person has been found unconscious, suspect an overdose, whatever the age. Do not be misled by the smell of alcohol into believing that the person is merely drunk—a large proportion of the tablets taken in overdose cases are washed down by alcohol. While considering other possible causes for coma, check out the possibility of overdose. Is there a note anywhere? Are there any empty pill bottles?

Staff receiving the patient in the accident and emergency department will appreciate information about what was taken, how much and when—all vital to the successful management of the patient. Wherever possible try to take the empty pill bottles with you.

Well-meaning attempts at making the patient sick should be discouraged. Giving salt water to drink is particularly dangerous as it may lead to a serious disturbance in the patient's blood chemistry, and cause vomiting later when the patient has become increasingly drowsy and may no longer be able to protect the airway. In addition, certain substances may do devastating damage to the respiratory tract—fumes from hydrocarbons such as petrol and spirits—or oesophagus—corrosive strong acids and alkalis—if vomiting is provoked. Drinking milk is a useful first aid measure in such cases as it provides a protective lining for the stomach.

Let patients talk if they wish. Do not moralise, or show resentment. These patients have problems, let them get these off their chest.

En route to hospital the patient may be concerned about having a stomach washout. This unpleasant, though not painful procedure is used to try to remove drugs from the patient's stomach before they can be passed into the gut and absorbed. A washout usually has to be performed within 6 h of the overdose if worthwhile amounts of the drug are to be recovered, although there are exceptions to this rule (see Table 13.2). The procedure consists of passing a wide-bore tube which the patient swallows into the stomach and then gently syphoning water in and out of the stomach to remove tablet debris.

Medicines to induce vomiting (such as syrup of ipecacuanha) are usually given to small children who have accidentally taken some tablets in mistake for sweets. A larger dose may be given to adults, provided that they are sufficiently conscious to protect their airway.

Difficult as patients who have indulged in self-harming behaviour may be, they are still patients in a potentially life-threatening condition and therefore deserve the fullest standards of professional care.

SELF-INFLICTED INJURY

Hawton and Catalan (1982), from their detailed 4-year study in Oxford, report a lack of suicidal intent in most cases. Of the 617 cases studied between 1976 and 1980, 80% consisted of lacerations to the wrists or forearm and a further 7% involved wounding elsewhere on the body. There was an overall female to male ratio of 3:2.

Self-inflicted injury tends to be a repeating pattern of behaviour, so you may well find that the person has multiple old scars. The wounds, however, are usually relatively superficial and it is very unusual for any deep structures to be involved. The patients will often feel no pain during the actual wounding, rather they feel a great tension building up inside them, which cutting relieves.

Deliberate self-harm presents emergency personnel with many problems. The person is often upset and may be uncooperative; other involved persons can range from being sympathetic and supportive to being aggressive and threatening. When the extent of the likely damage to the person appears small, and he or she is being difficult, it is easy to think 'What am I doing here? Is this what the ambulance service is for?' These are understandable feelings, but they will not help the situation, the patient or yourself. Any hostility on your part may provoke an attack, and will certainly not help to calm down the situation. Try to remove whatever was used to inflict the wounds by persuasion, never force, and move the patient voluntarily to the accident and emergency department for wound dressing and assessment.

References

Barraclough B. *et al.* (1974) A hundred cases of suicide; clinical aspects, *British Journal of Psychiatry*; **125**: 355–373.

Farmer R., Hirsch S. (1979) *The Suicide Syndrome*, London: Croom Helm.

Hawton K., Catalan J. (1982) *Attempted Suicide*. Oxford: Oxford Medical Publications.

Hospital In-patient Enquiry (1977) London: HMSO.

Morgan H. G. (1979) *Death Wishes? The Understanding and Management of Self-harm*. Chichester: John Wiley.

Tuckman J., Youngman W. F. (1968) A scale for assessing suicide risk for attempted suicide. *Journal of Clinical Psychology*, **24**: 17–19.

Walsh M. H. (1982) Patterns of drug overdose. *Nursing Times* **78**: 275–278.

Walsh M. H. (1985) *Accident and Emergency Nursing, A New Approach*. London: Heinemann.

14. Alcohol and Drug-related Problems

INTRODUCTION

Emergency personnel are having to cope with a steady increase in the numbers of patients whose problems are wholly or partly related to the use of drugs. The rights and wrongs of drug use are controversial, and it is not the place here to enter into a moral debate. However, remember the next time you are called to attend people who have collapsed with a possible heart attack, that their illness is probably the result of drug abuse, namely tobacco, an addictive drug responsible for many tens of thousands of deaths per year.

For various reasons, some drugs are socially acceptable and others are not, a fundamental concept in understanding drug use and abuse. What is more socially acceptable than a pint of beer? Yet it is estimated that there are 700 000 problem drinkers in the United Kingdom, of whom some 200 000 are addicted, while the cost to the nation of alcohol abuse is of the order of £1000 million per year (Paton, 1982). However, other drugs such as cannabis and heroin are socially unacceptable, their use defined as abuse and illegal, and the person using them seen either as a criminal or at best as sick. However, in other societies cannabis or the derivatives of the opium poppy are freely available, and again we see societies where fearful penalties are attached to the use of alcohol.

The answer to the question 'what is a drug-related problem' largely depends where you are in history and in which part of the world you are. There is no absolute right and wrong.

ALCOHOL-RELATED PROBLEMS

It is commonly thought that alcohol is a stimulant; it is not, it is a depressant. In moderate quantities inhibitions are removed, hence the more expansive, social behaviour associated with alcohol use. However, judgement and coordination are impaired while the normal inhibitions that tend to restrain us from behaving in an aggressive manner are diminished. The more alcohol consumed, the more dangerous the person becomes behind the wheel of a car, and the more prone to aggressive outbursts or other forms of unsociable behaviour. In large quantities alcohol causes drowsiness, diminished levels of consciousness and finally coma.

Alcohol and Violence

Experienced ambulance crew will have noticed the linkage between alcohol and violent behaviour. This is well illustrated by Honkanen (1975), who showed that in a major hospital, of persons involved in fights or who had inflicted deliberate self-harm on themselves, 86% had a positive blood alcohol level. Apart from conditions such as cirrhosis of the liver and major gastrointestinal bleeds, alcohol can be associated with assaults, road traffic accidents (drunken pedestrians as well as drunken drivers), social breakdown and ultimately vagrancy.

If summoned to people who have been involved in assaults a careful approach is needed as they will already be in an aggressive frame of mind (see p.148), and wrong cues from you will lead to possible further violence, particularly if alcohol is involved, due to removal of inhibitions. If they are heavily under the influence of alcohol, their ability to reason and remember will be impaired, so in talking to them keep it simple and do not become frustrated if you do not make much progress.

It is probably best to distance yourself from them, do not become emotionally involved in the situation, and if you meet with no cooperation after simple explanations of what is involved, then withdraw. The alternative is probably frustration, anger and possibly violence. The old adage about not arguing with a drunk is wise advice. Leave it to the police.

Alcohol and Head Injuries

Alcohol can greatly confuse the picture in the case of a person suffering from a head injury. Is the person's diminished level of consciousness due to the effects of the blow on the head or the alcohol? This is one of the most difficult problems to handle in the emergency field, for if you get it wrong, the person may suffer serious brain damage or die because no action was taken. Head injury is further complicated by the increased risk of vomiting in cases where the person has drunk large quantities. Indeed, it is possible for people to drink themself into a coma, vomit, and die from asphyxiation as a result of inhaling vomitus. Always remember the increased risk of vomiting when handling persons who appear to have consumed large quantities of alcohol.

A common situation for emergency personnel is to find people either unconscious or very drowsy, a smell of alcohol and some signs of head or facial trauma, such as matted blood in the hair or a facial wound. Nobody is able (or willing) to give an account of what happened or how long they have been in this state. They could be simply drunk, and have sustained a minor laceration in falling over, or have suffered a significant brain injury from their fall, or been assaulted in which case the risk of brain injury is that much greater. However, it is impossible to disentangle the effects of the alcohol from any trauma that may have occurred. The safest course of action is to assume that people have a significant head injury until proven otherwise, and therefore transfer them to the nearest accident and emergency unit with whatever information you can gather at the scene. In transit, manage patients as with any other head injury, and resist at all times the temptation to think of them as just a drunk. The true circumstances may be very different.

The Alcoholic

An alternative scenario that sometimes develops involves being called out to people under the influence of alcohol, who admit freely to being alcoholics and who state that they want medical treatment to help with their problems. However, while the psychiatric services will try to help alcoholics, the latter have to be sober when they ask for help, and therefore have full insight into what they are asking for and what is involved in treatment—this is usually lacking in someone under the influence of alcohol.

As there is a high potential for aggression in this situation, the best course of action is to suggest that alcoholics contact their general practitioner when sober, giving reasons. However, this may not be possible, and if they insist on being taken to the accident and emergency unit, this is probably the safest thing to do, even though there is little the unit can do except repeat the same advice.

Alcohol is likely to be present in many settings with which emergency personnel have to deal. It is wise, therefore, to approach such situations with caution and keep a low profile as an unguarded word can lead to a great deal of trouble. It is undesirable to have persons in the back of an ambulance still drinking. A basic ground rule should be that patients leave their bottles behind: 'You can come but your bottle can't', is the best line.

Management in Alcohol-related Problems

If a group of people is involved, only allow one to accompany the patient. The risk of aggression and violence from a group is greater than from a single person not only during transit, but subsequently in the accident and emergency unit. One of the prime reasons for this enhanced risk is that group responsibility for the consequences of any violent act is shared leading to reduced individual guilt. There is a desire to show off in front of an audience and members of the group encourage each other to go further in defying authority. It is easy to rationalise violence by saying it was only done to help the group, 'I only did it for my mates.' A group of people, especially when under the influence of alcohol, has a greater potential for trouble than any one individual. It is always a good policy therefore to remove patients from the group, allowing perhaps one person, preferably the quietest, to accompany them to hospital.

If members of the group insist on accompanying their friend, the simple answer is that the ambulance does not move until they get off. If they still refuse to leave the vehicle, summon the police, but do not become involved in conflict yourself. If force and threats are used to compel you to take the group with the patient, radio ahead so that the police may be waiting at the accident and emergency unit to deal with the troublemakers. But at all costs, try not to give way to pressure and allow a rowdy group of people who have been drinking to accompany the patient, or you will cause major problems both for yourself and subsequently for the accident and emergency staff.

OTHER FORMS OF DRUG USE
AND ABUSE

As we mentioned above, the definition of drug abuse is a social one, and therefore varies from society to society and from age to age.

At present, there is a marked increase in the quantities of drugs being used in the United Kingdom, and persons suffering from the harmful effects of their use are being dealt with more and more often by the emergency services. It is therefore worth briefly outlining the effects of the more common drugs encountered. It should be remembered that they are used in a wide variety of settings, and emergency personnel should therefore avoid the trap of thinking only of some sleazy cellar in a rundown inner city area as the haunt of drug users! From prosperous suburbia to council estates, the north of England to London (and particularly Edinburgh in Scotland), the potential is there for persons with drug-related problems.

Heroin

Heroin is also known on the street as scag, smack, H, horse etc. Much has been made recently of the problem of heroin addiction. Yet alcohol and tobacco kill tens of thousands of people a year, compared to maybe 200 or 300 who die as a result of heroin abuse, although it is assuming new importance due to its role in the spread of AIDS via contaminated needles.

However, there is no disguising the seriousness of the problem and the fact that it is growing. Heroin produces a euphoric effect when injected intravenously, which is the most common route used in the United Kingdom. It can also be inhaled or snorted (the common practice in Vietnam among American servicemen, most of whom returned home without becoming addicted). Like most drugs it requires a progressively larger dose to produce the same effect, which leads the user to ever bigger demands and the risk of accidental overdose.

There is some controversy about just how addictive heroin is. Psychological, social and physiological factors play a large part. The process of withdrawal from heroin addiction involves what is usually known as 'cold turkey'; the person experiences nausea and vomiting, abdominal pain, a rapid pulse, headaches and sweating. Within a couple of weeks physiological dependence on the drug is largely diminished, yet the relapse rate amongst addicts who have had their drugs withdrawn for this period, and then been released from an addiction centre remains near 100%, indicating the complex interplay of social and psychological factors.

Accidental Overdose

The first problem likely to be encountered by emergency personnel is a drug user who has accidentally overdosed. The effects of heroin and related narcotics (such as morphine or pethidine) include respiratory depression and coma; death from respiratory arrest is a strong possibility. The patient will be found with very shallow breathing, or even in a state of respiratory arrest, unable to be roused. Friends may be present who can give a history of heroin use, although they may be reluctant to do so for fear of legal repercussions. It is important to try to allay such fears; they must feel able to trust you if you are to obtain accurate information about what has been taken, how much, by what route, and when.

Signs that should alert you to the possibility of a narcotics overdose include pinpoint pupils, coma in the absence of alcohol or any other obvious reason such as a head injury or diabetes, and evidence of injection sites. Physical evidence to watch for obviously includes needles and syringes, but beware accidental inoculation with such high-risk items. Look out also for small pieces of aluminium foil, lying around, as illegal heroin is usually sold packaged in this way.

The first priority is to clear the airway and oxygenate the patient. Ventilation with a bag and oxygen supply may be needed if breathing is very shallow or has ceased; consider intubation if necessary. *Caution:* At this stage you must protect yourself due to the risks of hepatitis B and AIDS, both of which are bloodborne infectious diseases associated with illegal heroin users. Both blood and saliva are infective, so avoid introducing either into your own body by sensible precautions such as wearing a sticking plaster over any cut while on duty, and the use of disposable gloves.

The patient must be moved as quickly as possible to an accident and emergency unit, and resuscitated with the drug naloxone (Narcan), a specific antagonist to any narcotic, in the usual dose of 4 mg i.v., repeated if necessary; this will bring the patient around very quickly. Provided that you keep the patient well oxygenated en route to the hospital, a good recovery may be made in a remarkably short time.

Complications of Use

The second group of problems associated with illegal drug use involves the effects of dirty, shared needles and syringes and poor injection technique. Hepatitis B and AIDS have already been mentioned, and septicaemia, grossly infected injection sites, and even gangrene requiring amputation, are just some of the other complications of illegal i.v. drug use.

It is important to remember not to be judgemental about drug addicts. They have a range of serious problems, both medically and psychosocially. Basically they are not criminals or evil people, although their addiction may drive many of them to commit crime to raise money for drugs. Such crime might be avoided if they were treated as people in need of help rather than as criminals, as used to be the case in the late 1960s and early 1970s in the United Kingdom.

Hallucinogenics

Lysergic acid diethylamide (LSD) is the best-known drug in this group. Others include the so-called magic mushrooms which contain psylocybin as their active ingredient, but their effect is much less potent than LSD. A very powerful agent that so far has not made a widescale appearance in the United Kingdom is 'angel dust' (phencyclidine or PCP).

The effect of these drugs is to induce hallucinations and strange sensations such that users may feel colours or see sounds. Behaviour may become very deranged and bizarre, so much so that they are a danger to themselves and others. LSD is taken as small tablets usually in a group so that anybody experiencing a particularly 'bad trip' may be talked down by others in the group. The emergency services may be called if the situation gets out of hand.

Under the effect of a hallucinogenic, patients have little perception of reality, they may be unable to judge distances or sensations properly, they may even be very disturbed and violent. For their own protection they need restraint and sedation until the effects of the drug have worn off. If their colleagues cannot supply this, then the only recourse you have is to the police, a very unpopular step with those present for obvious reasons, but friends are usually of help. Removal to the accident and emergency department for sedation is essential, but remember that only the police are legally allowed to use force.

Due to the unpredictability of the effects of LSD, and also changing fads and trends, the drug is much less in evidence than it used to be in its heyday during the psychodelic, swinging 60s. But the fact remains that if you are called to a person who is on a bad trip as a result of LSD it is a serious emergency and should be treated as such.

Cannabis

When cannabis (also known on the street as hash, pot, marijuana, shit, grass, leb etc) is smoked it produces a feeling of mild euphoria, and little else. It is extremely unlikely that you would be called out to somebody using cannabis alone.

Amphetamines and Tranquillisers

Amphetamines (also known as uppers, speed and bennies) are popular among younger drug users. They are stimulants and the feeling of excitement and activity that they produce can be greatly enhanced by injecting the drug intravenously. A 'speed freak' may go for several days without sleep before 'crashing out' at the end of a 'run'. While under the influence of speed, a person may behave very erratically, show signs of mania, and be very aggressive, so caution is urged.

When called to deal with a young person who has been seen to be behaving in a disturbed manner, emergency personnel should consider drug use, most probably amphetamines, as a possible cause. Barbiturates and other tranquillising drugs (downers) may also be used with amphetamines, sometimes injected intravenously. All the risks of i.v. drug use discussed above also apply to this group.

Solvent Abuse

The use of inhaled drugs for recreation goes back as far as the 18th century when the likes of Coleridge, Southey and Wedgwood were reported as indulging in this practice. In modern times we are all familiar with the term 'glue-sniffing'. This is, in fact, misleading as virtually any organically based solvent can be used (such as hair spray, polystyrene cement, oven cleaners, petrol etc.), as can the propellants from aerosols (freons).

The effects are similar to alcohol in that the person suffers intoxication, a feeling of elation, unsteady gait, lack of coordination and may eventually become drowsy and comatose. The age group most affected are adolescents, males far more so than females.

Signs to look for when summoned to a collapsed adolescent are the smell of the substance on the breath, evidence of the material used lying around or in pockets, plastic bags or crisp packets used to inhale from, and redness around the mouth or nose. Chronic users often have sores.

The effects start to wear off after 30 minutes or so, when the person will start to recover consciousness, albeit in a rather confused state. Care of the airway in transit is the main priority; many deaths that have occurred have been due to airway problems.

In assessing the possibility of a case of solvent abuse, it is worth noting that cases have been reported from both ends of the social spectrum. Solvent abuse, like other forms of drug use, is not confined to poor rundown inner city areas.

Cocaine

Cocaine (alternative street names coke, snow, C etc.) is a stimulant, producing feelings of wellbeing and euphoria. It is known as the Rolls Royce of the drug world, and is generally held to be the most desirable drug to use due to its effects and the fact that it does not require i.v. injection and is therefore free from all the complications that go with this type of drug use. As a stimulant it produces raised blood pressure and pulse rate in users, the effects of a snort lasting about 30 minutes, so repeated use is needed to maintain a high. Ambulance personnel may encounter the term 'crack' which is slang for a very addictive pure crystalline form of cocaine. It is unlikely that emergency personnel will be called out to deal with a case of cocaine abuse.

CONCLUSIONS

One final point is worth making in connection with handling all patients where drug abuse is suspected. Your job is to look after an ill person, you are not a representative of the police drug squad. The trust of those present is vital if you are to gain their cooperation and the information you need to care for that patient to the best of your ability. Your principal responsibility is therefore to the patient, whose trust you must earn and keep.

References

Honkanen R. (1976) *Annals Chirurgiae et Gynaecologiae*, **65**: 282–287.
Paton A. (1982) Alcohol problems. London: *British Medical Journal*.

15. Communication and Organisation

INTRODUCTION

This chapter is divided into two parts: the first part is concerned with communication of all kinds: written and radio mainly, and liaison with other services; the second part deals with organisational planning for major events, riots and civil disturbances.

WRITTEN COMMUNICATION

All communication is important, and none more so than the written word. Patients taken into hospital after a doctor's visit will usually have a letter from the doctor. Ambulance crew should take charge of this letter, as it will usually contain vital information for the medical staff at the hospital. A good way of ensuring that it arrives safely is to make a habit of placing it on the stretcher once patients are loaded into the ambulance and leaving it there until they are handed over.

If patients are unable to give clear and reliable information (as, for example, a confused elderly patient from a nursing home) ask a relative (or member of staff in the case of an institution) to write down brief personal and medical details (such as medication taken). This information will greatly assist accident and emergency staff later. Do not assume that whoever accompanies patients will know a great deal about them as often they do not. If any information of use in contacting relatives can be obtained it should be recorded and passed on to accident and emergency staff later. When dealing with head injured patients or those who have taken overdoses etc., try to obtain their details from friends or relatives before leaving the scene. A patient may refuse to give them to you or may lapse into unconsciousness before you can get them.

Many ambulance services have a patient information form to record details concerning both the patient's condition and treatment given. If this is clear and concise it will provide a vital yardstick for hospital staff to measure the patient's progress. If this information is not recorded at the time, it may have been forgotten by the time it is needed. It is also important for the development of advanced skills that accurate records be kept of instances where crew have used these skills and to what effect.

RADIO COMMUNICATION

Ambulances are fitted with two-way radio to enable Control to maintain ready contact with other vehicles and vice versa. Crew should therefore ensure that they use their radio as effectively as possible. Control, the centre of the system, is usually a fixed transmitting and receiving station. The vehicles on the road are known as *mobiles*.

The system operates on VHF, and is designed in such a way that messages incoming to Control are only received by Control and not by any other mobiles. On an open channel system, therefore, all mobiles can always hear Control, but not normally each other. However, Control does have a talk-through facility, which if activated allows mobiles to speak to each other direct or to the local accident and emergency unit assuming it has a receiver fitted.

To facilitate identification, each control or mobile has its own call sign. To make a transmission, you start with the call sign of the mobile or Control that is to receive the message, then state your own call sign followed by the word 'over' to indicate you have finished and are awaiting a reply. The receiving mobile or Control identify themselves using the phrase 'go ahead, over' as the cue for you to state your message. All communication should be ended by Control with the phrase 'Control out' or 'Control standing by' which indicates they are available for any further message. This should not be confused with the term 'stand by' which means that Control want you to remain ready on your radio for further communication. When an urgent message needs to be passed on open channel sets, the term 'priority message' should always be used when calling Control.

Radios may be single-channel or multi-channel, the latter indicating that there are other frequencies available, used by other services. It is wise to find out what other services are tuned in on the different frequencies on your set to avoid confusion.

Emergency Reserve Channel (ERC)

The ambulance service has available the emergency reserve channel (ERC), which is literally that—a channel reserved for emergency transmission, not for everyday use. Controls all over the country monitor this channel so provided that you are within radio range, you can always contact a Control in the event of an emergency or some unexpected difficulty. For example, a mobile from Avon that was in Devon, could still get in touch immediately even if the crew did not know the Devon Control channel number, by turning to ERC and broadcasting 'Devam Control, Devam Control, this is Avam 3002, an Avon County Mobile, calling you on ERC, do you receive? Over.'

Reception and transmission can be difficult in certain locations because of natural or man-made obstacles such as mountains or buildings. If reception is poor or even non-existent, try a different location. Moving to a higher location will often help reception.

Open and Closed Systems

Some systems are simple open-channel systems where crew just pick up a microphone and can call Control at once. More advanced systems are computerised and closed, in other words, you need to press a button first to open the channel. When you press the call button on the set, your vehicle number is entered on a VDU at Control. A tone will sound on your radio to tell you that the call has been received. A stacking system if operating will store calls in the order they come in, ready for Control to reply. You must wait for a response as this may not be immediate at busy times. There will also be a priority button that allows you in an emergency to over-ride other calls and move to the top of the stack in Control with your call. Advanced systems such as these may also incorporate a pager that emits a bleeping sound when you are called, and is to be carried by crew when away from the vehicle as a means of informing them that Control is trying to make contact.

Pip Tones and Test Calls

Other radio systems use a pip tone: when another mobile is transmitting to control your hear pips coming over the radio. Calling control at the same time as another mobile may interfere with their message, so to avoid wasting time, wait for the pips to finish indicating that no other transmissions are being made, before proceeding with your own.

Test calls may be made to assess reception; the following convention is used to describe the quality of such a call.

Strength 1 : signal unreadable due to background noise
Strength 2 : signal barely readable due to background
Strength 3 : signal readable, background present
Strength 4 : signal good, slight background
Strength 5 : signal good, no background.

Squelch Control

If your radio is fitted with a squelch control, turning the knob on until interference is heard and then back, just until it disappears, will give you the optimum signal at maximum range.

Transmitting

When you are transmitting, be brief and precise. Think out your message in advance to avoid wasting time. If you are asking Control to relay a message to the hospital remember that the longer the message, the greater the chance of error creeping in. Avoid slang terms, they are both unprofessional and may lead to misunderstanding as they may mean different things to different people. An accident and emergency unit on standby for you should have an estimated time of arrival (ETA) if you are taking in a serious case.

When using the microphone talk slowly, clearly and across it but ensure your mouth is close to it. The words affirmative and negative should be used for yes and no. To acknowledge receipt of a message terms such as 'Roger' (message received), or 'Wilco' (message received and I will comply) are used.

To spell out words use the standard international phonetic alphabet as follows (if you are using figures, prefix them with the word 'figures'):

A : Alpha	J : Juliet	S : Sierra
B : Bravo	K : Kilo	T : Tango
C : Charlie	L : Lima	U : Uniform
D : Delta	M : Mike	V : Victor
E : Echo	N : November	W : Whiskey
F : Foxtrot	O : Oscar	X : X-Ray
G : Golf	P : Papa	Y : Yankee
H : Hotel	Q : Quebec	Z : Zulu
I : India	R : Romeo	

Note also that the number 0 is always called zero. Correct use of the radio is vital to emergency personnel in the field, as careless usage is unprofessional and leads to mistakes and misunderstanding.

LIAISON WITH OTHER SERVICES

We have seen elsewhere (see p. 159) that first impressions are very important in determining how we perceive people. If ambulance personnel are to work well with representatives of the other services, it follows that they should seek to create a favourable first impression (they should also strive to maintain that impression by the excellence of their work subsequently!).

Fortunately, there is a high degree of commitment to the service, and because of this, the ambulance service has already achieved a high degree of professionalism, despite the lack of government resources with which it has had to contend. A well-organised, professional approach is a major asset in creating that vital first impression that will help gain the cooperation of both the general public and the other services. An integral part of this approach is to make sure that your uniform is correct and smartly turned out. Make sure you can be identified as ambulance crew, and remember the fluorescent jackets labelled

'Ambulance' are supplied to be worn at all RTAs for your own protection as much as anything else, so wear them!

Your approach should be calm and logical; this ensures that you get your priorities in the right order, gain control of the situation, and as we have seen (p. 149) helps calm everything down. So, having started off on the right foot by creating a good professional image, what next?

Police and Fire Brigade

A good rule of thumb is to remember that the police are in overall charge of the incident, the fire brigade are in charge of any environmental hazards such as fire or chemical leakage, and *you*

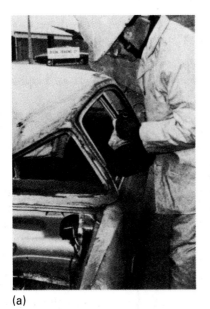 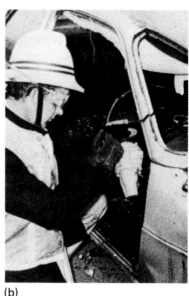

(a)   (b)

Fig. 15.1   (a) and (b) A power-operated abrasive cutting disc being used to cut through a structural member. Note the hand and eye protection afforded to the operator to supplement his normal operational uniform

are in charge of the patient. Normally both the other two services will be only too happy to let you get to the patient, they usually have enough problems of their own. If there are any difficulties of patient access, a firm but polite request such as 'Excuse

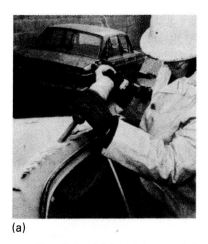 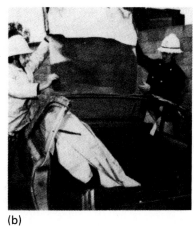

(a)   (b)

Fig. 15.2   (a) A compressed air operated cutting tool removing a
section of roof. (b) A roof section being removed after cutting

me, but can I get to the patient?' will usually be all that is
required.

You must ensure that you check the patient as soon as you
arrive on scene (bearing in mind the need for caution in the case
of chemical incidents etc.), especially in the case of a patient who
is trapped. The patient's condition must be stabilised and, if possible, blood samples taken and an infusion started so that deterioration can be prevented during the period they are trapped.
Having done this, try to get the blood samples off to the receiving
hospital as quickly as possible so that whole blood can be made
ready for your arrival. The patient's condition must be monitored at intervals to assess if there is any deterioration. If this
means asking the rescuers to stop work briefly then that is what
you must do. The criterion is to get the patient out in the best
possible condition for recovery, and not necessarily in the short-
est possible time. Remember also that if anyone is to stay with
the patient it should be you. Do not forget to send for an officer
from your own service if you consider it is necessary.

If you need assistance from other personnel on scene, a polite
request to the senior officer on site will usually be all that is
needed. If patients are being extricated from wreckage, ambulance crew must work closely with the fire brigade. (Figs. 15.1,
15.2 and 15.3). Do not be afraid to advise, and if you feel what is
being proposed is harmful, say so. When moving the patient with

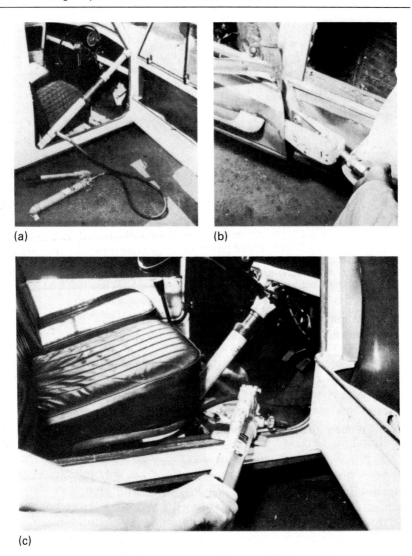

(a)   (b)

(c)

Fig. 15.3   (a) A partially extended hydraulic ram in position. (b) A hydraulic attachment ideal for use in small openings. (c) A hydraulic ram in position against a steering column

other helpers make sure that you take control and organise them properly. Uncoordinated action can only harm the patient.

Following a road traffic accident (RTA) the police may wish to breathalyse the patient or may ask you to wait for some reason.

If the condition of the patient is sufficiently serious to warrant removal to hospital immediately then you are the one to make that decision, not the police. First explain to them that they must see the patient at the hospital, and then move.

Officers of the other services should be treated with respect, but not deference. Ambulance personnel are the specialists in their own field and as such have responsibility for patient care. Officers of the other services will almost always be cooperative if they see you are professional and reasonable in your approach. If, however, there is a problem and you are denied access to the patient, ambulance crew should inform the relevant officer that they hold him responsible for this. Any harm the patient comes to as a result will be his responsibility, ask his name and tell him that a report on the incident will be submitted to the chief ambulance officer. Having said this, cooperation is generally good, and with a professional, positive approach, it is hoped that onsite relationships will go from good to even better.

Cave and Mountain Rescue Teams

A patient who is trapped underground or on a high crag presents a special set of problems as a specialist cave or mountain rescue team may be involved. They will have skills that you may not, skills that may be essential to reach the patient safely. The important thing is to ensure that you have access to the patient as quickly as possible to stabilise his or her condition. At times it may therefore be better to wait for the patient to be brought to you by the rescue team.

Emergency personnel should establish what are the rescue team's plans, and at what stage they can gain access to the patient. Mountain rescue teams are extremely proficient, but the paramedic may possess skills not available to the team, so even if you cannot accompany them, try to maintain a radio link so that you can offer advice during the rescue.

Major accident and emergency units are capable of supplying a mobile medical team that can supplement the resources of the ambulance team if required. They will be able to offer intravenous analgesia with powerful drugs such as diamorphine, facilities for onsite anaesthesia and surgical expertise. It is a mistake to wait until the trapped patient's condition has deteriorated before calling out the team as a last resort. The paramedic should get an early estimate from the fire brigade or rescue team of how long release or rescue might take, assess the patient's injuries and condition, and make a decision about the need for a hospital team. It is better to get the team out and find they are not needed than to call them late and leave them with a moribund patient for whom they can do nothing. There are occasions when the only way to release a patient is amputation of the trapped limb; the sooner this is done the better for the patient's survival.

When en route to the accident and emergency unit with a seriously injured patient, radio ahead giving ETA and a brief summary of the patient's injuries. This will be greatly appreciated by the accident and emergency unit and allows early mobilisation of resources at the hospital such as opening up a theatre ready for emergency surgery, contacting senior medical staff etc.

On arrival, emergency personnel should remember the advice on p. 159 concerning their manner and how first impressions do count. Professional handover of the patient with all the relevant information is required, conducted out of earshot of the patient, who may be a lot more aware of what is happening than you think; there is no point in causing extra stress.

One final word about liaison with other services in the field concerns the medical profession. If doctors are present, they take legal responsibility for the patient's wellbeing. However, in the case of an accident, it is unlikely that the doctor will be an expert in the field of trauma, and even less likely that he or she will have any experience of handling casualties in the field, unless a member of BASICS, the British Association of Immediate Care Schemes. If this organisation is active in your area, efforts should be made to develop a good liaison with its members as it is capable of supplying valuable medical expertise in the field. However, ambulance crew should not abdicate their responsibility for the patient simply because there is a doctor present. They must ensure that the best possible treatment is given.

MAJOR DISASTER PLANNING

It is impossible to define precisely what constitutes a major disaster, but, for planning purposes, the following should be taken into consideration: the number of casualties; severity and type of injury; involvement of other emergency services; and finally, whether the health authority has sufficient resources to cope on its own.

Given that it is impossible to define a major disaster in advance, the emergency services are in the position of having to wait for the event to happen, and then declaring it a major disaster in order that the full plan may be activated. It is therefore the responsibility of a senior officer of either the police, fire brigade or ambulance service to declare the incident a major disaster.

All ambulance services have a major disaster plan with which personnel should be familiar. Ideally it should be carried on each front-line vehicle.

Planning Principles

It is absolutely essential that everybody on site knows who is in charge, therefore overall control will rest with police, and their police control vehicle will be designated the *incident control centre*, identified by a blue and white chequered flag. The ambulance service and fire brigade will need their own control vehicles close by incident control, but it must be emphasised that while ambulance crew work under their own control, overall responsibility rests with the police. Identification of control vehicles may be helped by a rule that only they will display flashing blue lights on site.

Development of an Incident

Let us now consider how an incident may develop. The first ambulance crew on site have a major responsibility, not the obvious one of giving care to the injured, but that of gaining and passing on information. If this is not done as speedily and accurately as circumstances permit, there may be fatal delays in activating the major disaster plan and mobilising sufficient resources to deal with casualties.

The driver of the first vehicle on scene must establish and maintain radio contact with Control and pass on the following information:

(1) Details of what can be seen from the vehicle.
(2) Exact location and extent of the incident.

(3) Casualty estimate as seen from the vehicle.
(4) What other services are present.
(5) Any environmental hazards, such as fire, toxic fumes.

The attendant meanwhile should investigate the incident (bearing in mind safety) with the express purpose of discovering as much information as possible as quickly as possible. Hard though it may be, they should not at this stage become involved in casualty care as information is needed by Control urgently. They should assess:

(1) the scale and extent of the incident;
(2) the best access to and from site;
(3) the best estimate of casualties together with numbers trapped;
(4) the hazards on site, fire, fumes, flooding etc;
(5) the specialist services needed, such as gas board, armed services etc.

Ambulance Control need all this information quickly from the scene as this is the basis on which they will have to decide whether to declare the incident a major disaster. If Control takes this decision, they will usually have to initiate the following actions immediately.

(1) Dispatch a station officer to the scene as incident officer.
(2) Dispatch a radio car or mobile control to site (VHF and UHF).
(3) Contact police and fire brigade to check they are fully aware of events.
(4) Put designated hospitals on standby and confirm major disaster status as soon as possible.
(5) Request mobile medical teams from designated hospitals.
(6) Mobilise resources and personnel within ambulance service.
(7) Dispatch the equipment vehicle.
(8) Contact specialist services as needed, such as the gas board.

Speed of mobilisation depends on the speed at which that first vehicle on site reports an accurate assessment of the situation back to Control, hence the importance of not getting diverted from your information gathering and communication role if you are the first on the scene.

Responsibilities of the Crew and Other Personnel

The crew of the first vehicle can start vital organisational work while awaiting the arrival of their colleagues and the ambulance incident officer. The driver must maintain radio contact at all times while the attendant looks for suitable ambulance parking points on firm ground and locations that can be used as casualty collecting points, casualty loading points (with turning space for vehicles) and equipment storage points. The attendant may also need to liaise with the other services present during this early phase and organise any first aiders present. Clearly they cannot do everything at once, so logical decisions about priorities are needed.

The responsibilities of subsequent crews arriving on scene can be summarised as follows:

(1) Always enter and leave by the designated route.

(2) Park in the ambulance area without obstructing access.

(3) Ensure that you know your role before arrival; personnel may be divided into those with advanced skills required at some parts of the scene, while other personnel may be allocated different responsibilities.

(4) The driver should stay with the vehicle maintaining radio silence, but ready to respond when called and move accordingly.

(5) The attendant should report arrival to incident Control.

(6) During casualty care and evacuation, use equipment on the vehicle, avoiding if possible taking equipment away from site stocks when moving casualties.

(7) On leaving the incident call main Control, reporting casualty numbers and type; they will direct you to the appropriate hospital.

(8) Report arrival at hospital to main Control.

(9) Ensure that paperwork is complete, a mundane but vital point in the confusion that may surround a major disaster.

(10) Return as quickly as possible, restocking from hospital.

(11) Contact the ambulance liaison officer at hospital before departure (or Control if necessary).

Personnel working at a major disaster must stay within an ordered framework. Uncoordinated, individual action can cause confusion and delay, being counterproductive in the long run. This must be balanced by flexibility on the part of those on site, for it is impossible to foresee exactly what will happen—if that were so, the disaster could have been prevented in the first place! Fortunately disasters are rare, which means personnel must keep up to date on local plans to fill in the details sketched out above. Know your disaster plan!

PLANNING FOR MAJOR EVENTS

Major events such as sports competitions and music festivals may involve many thousands of people for lengthy periods of time. Sports may be of a sufficiently dangerous nature such as powerboat or motorcar racing to alert the organisers to the need for an efficient and expert emergency service on site. However, a relatively harmless pastime such as kicking a football around should not need such elaborate emergency contingency planning—should it? Unfortunately the supporters of Bradford City or Juventus football clubs bear tragic testimony to the need for a well-organised emergency contingency plan at all major events.

The two most important aspects of organising a major event are preplanning and communication. Nothing should be left to the day itself; while if there is insufficient communication, chaos and confusion will be the result.

To this end, a working committee should be formed of people who will both carry out the work beforehand and help organise on the day. The responsibilities of each member should be clearly defined and the committee should meet regularly to update its members. A working coordinator should be appointed, who will have overall responsibility both through the planning stage and on the day. He or she must attend the committee meetings. One further important point that must not be overlooked is insurance cover for all those helping to provide the first aid support. On this foundation a major event can be built.

Preplanning

Preplanning should try to anticipate contingencies that may arise. A large-scale map of the site is essential, on which first aid points, ambulance parking positions and access routes can all be plotted. It will also permit easier liaison with other services that may be involved, such as the police. Covering the map by a clear sheet of perspex allows it to be drawn on, and changed freely as the day evolves.

The distribution of resources around the site, both materials and personnel, should be carefully planned. Where will the first aid centre be, and how will it be staffed and equipped, are crucial questions that need careful consideration. The sort of equipment needed will range from stretchers (including scoop and para-guard), blankets, waterproof sheeting, rescue tools, torches and lighting, through cardiac monitors, resuscitation equipment to bandages, paper towels, pens and paper. It should be remembered that none of this equipment is of any use if it is in the wrong place, or if there is nobody present who knows how to use it. Preplanning avoids that sort of mistake.

Communication

Both voluntary services' ambulances and NHS vehicles have their own radios. Communication should be established in advance between the local ambulance Control and the event first aid Control. In some instances it may be sensible to have a county ambulance service officer on duty at the event. The use of personal radios can give greater speed and flexibility in onsite communication, provided that a proper radio discipline is observed, and matters do not deteriorate into a CB 'free for all'. The communication centre should have immediate access to the event loudspeaker system.

A thorough briefing session is mandatory for all staff in the field, and a well-prepared site map will be worth its weight in gold at this point. Everyone should be briefed about his or her responsibilities, and given the opportunity to ask questions to clear up any uncertainties. A clear policy about moving patients to ambulances or the ambulances to patients should be laid down at the briefing. A copy of the site map with access routes, first aid posts, etc. should be issued to personnel at the briefing sessions. Finally, let your local accident and emergency unit know about the event, and any implications it may have for them.

PLANNING FOR RIOTS AND
CIVIL DISTURBANCES

Major riots in our urban areas have unfortunately become a fact of life in the 1980s. Policing methods have had to change to cope with this unfortunate development, and so too must ambulance methods.

The impartiality of the ambulance service should be its best defence, although this impartiality is not always recognised by an angry mob in a riot. To stand in a street surrounded by an angry mob with the police outnumbered by five to one, trying to move a patient whose injuries are alleged to have been caused by the police, while bottles fly over your head and smash against the side of the ambulance, is an experience not to be recommended.

Sometimes it is possible to anticipate the violence. An event such as a mass picket in a controversial industrial dispute is usually known about in advance and the police draw up their plans accordingly. The ambulance service can be incorporated into the plan. In this case the scene resembles a medieval battle with both sides lined up ready facing each other, and the ambulance service waiting to pick up the pieces. However, urban riots of the sort witnessed recently in areas like Toxteth, Liverpool or St Pauls, Bristol, tend to be much less predictable, and it only needs one flashpoint incident to ignite the riot. In the early stages the police have difficulty in controlling the situation due to the weight of numbers drawn up against them (in opposing the police, communications can be very efficient involving not just word of mouth and the telephone, but also citizens band radio to muster forces), and it is in this early stage of hostilities that serious casualties may occur. The follow on situation, which may continue over several days, can then be anticipated and plans drawn up to deal with it.

Contingency planning is therefore essential to try to gain control of the situation as early as possible, and the ambulance service is essential to such planning. Each situation is different, therefore hard and fast rules are not possible, rather flexible guidelines based on experience are offered here.

Guidelines for Riots

Initial Situations

The fundamental rule is that *the police, if present, are in charge.*

While they should respect your expertise and allow you to practise normally for as long as possible, if they tell the crew to pick up a patient and go immediately, or to move out of an area at once, then these instructions must be obeyed. Ambulance crew do not know what is happening in the next street or just around the corner, but the police do, so their instructions must be followed.

As a general rule, a riot situation demands that you use a scoop and run policy, both for your safety and for the patient's welfare. The ambulance provides a ready focus for a crowd to gather, and flashing blue lights in a dark street can easily be mistaken for a police vehicle, turning the ambulance into a potential target. Use of the ambulance siren can have the same unfortunate effect and is therefore to be discouraged.

A riot is no place for bravado; discretion is the better part of valour, and if confronted by a hostile crowd crew should not risk provoking aggression but withdraw quickly. Female ambulance personnel need to be particularly aware of the potential sexual harassment in such situations.

On approaching a situation which appears potentially dangerous, and at which there is no police presence, notify Control immediately and tell them what you can see from the vehicle. Request police assistance as quickly as possible and if you feel that the situation is too dangerous, withdraw until they arrive.

If staying at the scene, park the vehicle pointing away from the scene to ensure that you have an available exit route. To make sure that you are clearly recognised as ambulance personnel, wear the fluorescent jacket labelled 'Ambulance' and the hard white safety hat, as much for protection as identification. Leave the vehicle with doors closed, but make sure they are unlocked in case you need to make a speedy exit. Carry the keys with you *at all times*.

Ambulance crew should stay together as two people are less likely to be attacked than one. Try to get the crowd to help you in dealing with casualties; this will defuse the 'them and us' situation and help the crowd realise you are genuinely neutral. Remember the advice from Chapter 11 on psychology and adopt a low profile. Do not respond to any provocative taunts or gestures and avoid physical contact as far as possible. In the emotionally charged atmosphere of a street riot, one wrong move could be construed as an aggressive act and lead to violence directed at ambulance crew.

As far as possible ignore the odd missile that is thrown, unless of course it is very dangerous, even if it hits the ambulance. Never get drawn into arguments with the crowd, if this is how the situation is developing it is time to withdraw, informing the police accordingly. A useful step is to pull down the interior blinds on the ambulance to limited the effects of flying glass should a missile break a window.

It is a mistake to assume that the crowd see you as a neutral helper; they may become angry simply because you are there and see you as part of the establishment they are fighting. A tactful withdrawal can be followed later, when passions have cooled, by a helpful presence.

If you are about to withdraw from an ugly situation, consider any foot policemen who may be in danger. Enquire tactfully if they wish to come with you, if they do the driver should get in the vehicle first and start the engine, and only then should the attendant and police officers join them. You may lose your neutral status in the eyes of the crowd but, as events in Tottenham tragically showed, you may save a police officer's life.

If you are working at night always carry a torch with you, even when entering people's houses; if somebody throws the light switch suddenly, you still have a source of light available. Wherever possible you should keep Control informed of your movements.

Anticipated Situations

In anticipated situations most of the previous comments will apply, where appropriate, but normally plans would be drawn up to cope with the situation and ambulance staff taking part would be briefed as to their roles. Here you will be operating as part of a team and this is no place for uncoordinated individual action. Listen closely to the briefing and be sure that you understand your role.

Patient retrieval will probably consist of first aid parties, snatch squads or vehicles with more than two crew members. In this situation the driver of the vehicle should stay in the driving seat and leave the engine running whilst keeping a careful eye on proceedings.

Close radio contact with Control is essential throughout the incident so that they know not only where you are, but also that you are safe. The driver should report any major escalation of the incident to Control at once, as your vehicle may be the only representative of the emergency services on hand to witness what might be a dangerous and threatening development.

If ordered into an area with a police escort, stay close to the police and do not get separated. Be prepared for quick action. Act under their instructions at all times—the middle of a riot is no place for a debate. If you are a member of a forward first aid party or snatch squad stick to your colleagues like glue, it is your best protection.

The hospital turnround needs to be speedy after a quick, efficient evacuation. If a procedure is in place to take police casualties to a different accident and emergency unit from the rioters, adhere closely to this policy.

Be careful what you say to civilians present. They may be from the media and comments made at the height of the trouble may be regretted the next day, especially if they are in print and appear to distort the facts.

It is difficult for the ambulance service to appear impartial during a riot as such close liaison with the police is needed. However, this should be the aim and each casualty should be treated equally according to the severity of the injuries, regardless of which 'side' the casualty is on. If the community normally sees the ambulance service as a helpful, professional service free from prejudice and bias in the way it treats people, then in abnormal situations such as riots it will start off with a major advantage.

16. Handling the Patient on Site

INTRODUCTION

In this chapter we deal with problems presented by the location of the site itself, and then problems of moving the patient, and various ways of lifting and aids to transportation.

PROBLEMS PRESENTED BY THE SITE

The number of problems presented by the site is as infinite as the number of different sites. An open and flexible mind is therefore required, together with the ability to anticipate problems before they develop. However, beware the trap of rigidly sticking to a preconceived plan of action worked out en route. Be prepared to adapt your care to the circumstances on scene.

Finding the Site

One of your first problems is finding the scene of the call. A numbered house in a street is usually easy to find, but a location in a large industrial complex is a different matter. There may be several different gates, but in this case they will usually be numbered so make sure you have the number from Control before you arrive. Sports grounds, airports, docks and railway premises are all examples of large areas with multiple entrances where you need accurate directions to avoid wasting precious time trying to find the exact scene of the incident. If a guide can be waiting to meet you at the main entrance, so much the better. Locations in the countryside can be particularly difficult. Ensure that you obtain directions from Control, either from somewhere you know or from a point that you can identify on a map.

Other Emergency Services

Other information you need concerns what other emergency services are on site or on their way. When you arrive you may feel they are needed, and it only wastes time if you are attempting to call them when they are already responding and on their way. Do not hesitate to ask Control for any extra information that you think you may need to function effectively on site beyond the initial call. Control should have the resources to get the information for you. When you arrive on site, the first consideration should be one of safety. For both your patient's sake and your own, be aware and observant as you approach. Protect the scene—the patient and yourself. Do not become the next casualty.

Road Accidents

Tankers Carrying Dangerous Substances

Road traffic accidents involving tankers are not to be approached lightly. Tankers and lorries carrying dangerous substances should have a Hazchem or other warning sign detailing the substance involved or warning of its effects, although foreign vehicles may not (see Appendix A, p. 250). If in doubt, approach from the upwind direction so that any toxic fumes will be blowing *away* from you, and avoid contact with any substance that has escaped from the vehicle. If there is a spillage of liquid, park the ambulance uphill of the scene.

If you can get close enough to read the Hazchem sign, pass details on to Control who will in turn relay this information to the fire brigade if they are not yet on site. If the police have not been called, make sure they are as their presence is essential in what could be a potentially very dangerous situation. Crowd control and even evacuation may be needed. The police have overall control of the scene, but the fire brigade are in charge of the specific leakage or fire and have the responsibility for saying when it is safe to approach. *Smoking is clearly banned in the vicinity of such an incident.*

If the victims of the accident have suffered chemical injury, then it is essential to follow any special instructions related to the chemicals involved. Any advance warning you can give the hospital receiving the casualties will be greatly appreciated. Information necessary for the treatment of casualties affected by the substance carried can be obtained from Control (with Hazchem details), the driver of the vehicle and from a 'Tremcard' which is carried on the vehicle. Remember that a number of substances affect respiration, although this may not be immediately obvious.

Fire Hazards

If we look at road accidents in general, we should note that one of the major hazards (apart from other traffic, especially on motorways) is fire, due to the risk of petrol spillage from ruptured fuel tanks or lines. Fortunately the incidence of fire is not too common in RTAs, but can be devastating when it occurs. Extreme caution is needed if there is a petrol spillage; ensure that the car engine is switched off, and if the casualty is trapped disconnect the battery. Have your vehicle fire extinguisher standing by with the casualty until the fire brigade arrive, if they are not on scene already. A horrific fire can be ignited by a simple spark, smouldering electrical wiring, a hot exhaust pipe, or a bystander smoking.

Such is the fire hazard in many emergency situations, that personnel should be aware of the standard colour coding for the different type of fire extinguishers as listed below:

Red	Water: use for wood or paper fire, but not for electrical or petrol fire.
Cream	Foam: use for petrol, oil etc., not for electrical fires.
Blue	Dry powder: use for electrical, liquid or mechanical fires.
Black	Carbon dioxide: use for any fire.
Green	BCF (bromochlorodifluoromethane, a liquid under pressure): use for any fire.

Note: With dry powder carbon dioxide and BCF, caution must be exercised when using them in confined spaces due to their possible effect on respiration.

Moving Traffic

Moving traffic is a danger at all road accidents. Wear fluorescent jackets at all times for safety. Leave blue lights, four-way flashers and side-lights on at the scene, and rear fog lights on if foggy. The police may not appreciate the scale of the accident from the initial call, so check that they are on their way if you get there first.

Electricity Hazards

Electricity is another hazard with which to contend. Beware of overhead power lines that may be down, as well as power cables exposed at the site of the accident, for example, in a trench. Do *not* approach the casualty unless the electricity is switched off. This also applies under pylons and in substations.

Railways

Railways should be treated with caution, especially in these days of quiet, high-speed trains. Control should be notified immediately to make sure that the railway authorities have shut the lines to traffic and switched off power cables or third rails.

Building Sites

If the casualty is at a building site or quarry, check that work has been suspended in the vicinity. Watch out for half-covered holes or unstable workings that might lead to rockfalls etc.

Underground Sites

Underground locations have peculiar hazards of their own. Sewers or tunnels are dangerous because of the pockets of gas that may accumulate. Make sure you have an expert adviser with you, and attach a rope to the person going in after the casualty as an insurance policy. Naked lights must be avoided due to the explosion hazard (as was tragically shown at Abbeystead recently). Make sure the operation has been shut down and that those in charge are aware of people in the tunnel. If the tunnel is designed to carry water, the last thing rescue personnel want is a flash flood.

Caution: if the situation involves a suspected bomb, avoid using your radio in the vicinity as it may trigger certain devices; move well away or use the phone for communication.

Civil Disturbances

Civil disturbances in urban areas (see also Chapter 15, p. 216) are a new problem for ambulance personnel, who should not expect exemption from possible violence in these situations, so caution is advisable. If you arrive at a volatile situation, you should consider asking for police assistance before going in. If your vehicle is left unattended, make sure that you have the keys on you. If the situation seems unpredictable or menacing, make sure Control are aware of this, and if you go in to a patient always stay together with your colleague.

Domestic Incidents

Domestic incidents can present unpredictable hazards. Make sure you have found out all you can before entering the house, and be on your guard for the possibility that weapons may be involved, even firearms. Again, go in together. It may be necessary to call the police if you are refused entry.

Brawls

Another hazardous situation is being called out to the scene of a brawl involving a group of people, especially at night. As stated above, your role as a member of the emergency services gives you no protection against possible violence. Involve the police before you investigate if the situation looks at all dubious. Avoid standing in the middle of a group; for your own protection try to keep the group in front of you and have a wall at your rear—that way you will at least see trouble coming if matters deteriorate. Keep together and keep cool, remembering the advice in Chapter 11 on the psychological approach. A large torch is indispensable when attending calls at night as lighting may be very poor, especially in some of the less salubrious areas where this type of trouble may arise.

If patients are carrying a weapon do not turn your back on them. However, you should try to avoid eye-to-eye contact as it can be very provocative in this situation. Try to disarm them by

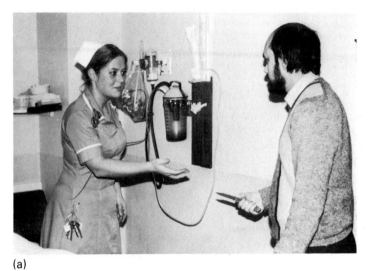

(a)

(b)

Fig. 16.1 The patient with a weapon. (a) The wrong approach: here the nurse has allowed the patient to get between her and the exit. She is holding out her hand demanding the knife and she is making eye-to-eye contact. This is confronting and threatening to the patient and may cause him to respond violently and he may use the knife to inflict serious harm. (b) The right approach. The nurse is keeping close to the exit and is asking the patient to place the weapon on neutral territory before attempting to remove it. She is keeping at a safe distance (arm's length) and avoiding eye-to-eye contact. (c) If attacked with a weapon you should try to smother it with a blanket or anything else available, while retreating rapidly to safety and calling for help

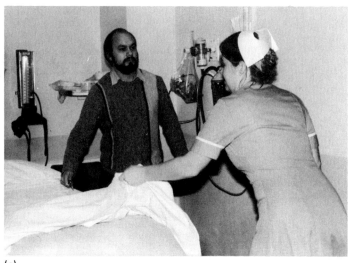

(c)

suggesting that they do not need the weapon, or to threaten you, as you are there to try to help. Ask them to place the weapon aside on neutral territory rather than give it directly to you; again this is less threatening and involves less loss of face. Suggest they put it on a table or some such surface, your strategy then being to try to manoeuvre them away from the weapon, or at least get it out of arm's reach (Fig. 16.1). Always exercise great caution and remember that the police have more expertise than you in this field, so if you can stall for time until they arrive this may be the best approach.

If you wear glasses remember to take them off *before* getting involved in a difficult situation. Taking them off in front of the patient is a clear cue that you expect violence, while leaving them on could result in serious eye damage if the situation worsens.

The importance of a cautious approach to the scene cannot be overemphasised. Emergency personnel will sometimes find themselves in hazardous situations. But remember that you are all the patient has got; if anything happens to you, it is the patient who will suffer.

WORKING ON SITE

We can now consider the problems that arise once you have safely got to the scene. A simple problem that may occur once you have located the scene is when the attendant is taken to the patient urgently while the driver parks the vehicle. The driver may then find that everybody has gone, and there is no way of finding the way to the patient due to a locked door or lack of adequate direction. If possible, leave someone to show the way.

Always ensure that you have your Brook airway in the first aid box. The information given may be inaccurate with the result that if you find yourself unexpectedly walking in on a cardiac arrest situation, the Brooks airway allows you to ventilate the patient without fear of catching any infectious disease while the bag and mask and other resuscitation equipment is fetched from the vehicle.

It is wise if both driver and attendant go to the patient initially, pooling their resources of knowledge and experience to assess both the situation and the patient. The driver can then return to the vehicle if necessary to collect any other equipment needed, while the attendant can commence treatment.

If you know there is likely to be a substantial journey to the patient, consider taking equipment with you that may be needed when you first arrive. It can easily be carried on the stretcher and can save you extra journeys. To save precious time, if a lift is required to reach the patient, get somebody to hold the lift for you or jam something in the door to hold it at your floor.

Look beyond the patient to the immediate environment. Substantial improvements may be possible just by asking somebody to turn something off or move equipment that is in your way. Try to clear bystanders away to give you the best working conditions. They may inadvertently cause you to lose your balance while lifting or moving the patient. Ask for more light if needed.

No two situations are ever the same. Ambulance crew should therefore be prepared to learn all the time. Think laterally: can equipment be used for other purposes than the obvious? One ambulance man rescued a patient from a cellar full of toxic fumes by using the portable oxygen resuscitator the ambulance carried as a breathing apparatus for himself. This enabled him to reach the patient, with whom he shared it while dragging the patient to safety. Another example is the jack your ambulance carries which will do many things besides allowing you to change a tyre on your own vehicle: it can greatly help stabilise wreckage when people are trapped and the fire brigade has yet to arrive, or even free them altogether.

It is also helpful to review the situation after the patient has been safely delivered to hospital. Could you have handled it differently? Only by being prepared to evaluate your actions and consider how effective they were will you progress and be that little bit wiser.

PATIENT MOVEMENT ON SITE

Having assessed your patient and arrived at a working idea of the main problems, there are then two major decisions to be made. Does the patient need moving, and if so, how?

When Moving the Patient is Unnecessary

Many patients can be effectively treated at the scene. Some calls to collapses turn out to be people who have merely fainted, and recover quickly after lying flat for a few minutes. If, however, the person is elderly every attempt should be made to persuade him or her to go to hospital as the cause of their apparent faint may be a disturbance in heart rhythm or a minor stroke temporarily affecting blood flow to the brain. Sometimes elderly patients fall out of bed and cannot get back. But once returned to bed, a worthwhile move is to advise relatives to get the person's general practitioner to check the patient over the following day. There are therefore simple situations which can be successfully resolved without moving the patient at all.

Calling Out the General Practitioner

If the patient's condition requires immediate treatment, over and above what the paramedic can give at the scene, they must be moved to hospital. However, if the illness is of a minor nature, or of a long-term nature which requires hospitalisation but not immediate treatment, it may well be more beneficial to arrange for their GP to call. This may save the patient a long wait in an A&E department (bearing in mind that the doctor may take some time to arrive). Put yourself in the patient's place but err on the side of caution.

Diabetic patients who become hypoglycaemic generally recover after being given 50 ml of 50% dextrose intravenously. Usually there is no need to move them to hospital but if the cause is not known it is wise to arrange for their GP to call before you leave.

The Best Way to Move the Patient

Assuming that we have decided to move the patient, the next question is how? It is possible to calculate that in an average career, ambulance crew will have to move something like 300 000 patients. The implication of this figure is that if you wish to avoid serious back injury you only lift when you have to, and then do so very carefully! Many patients can walk to the ambulance themselves, perhaps with an arm to steady them if they are elderly—for example, patients with arm or wrist injuries, or some with back pain who cannot bend. All patients do not have to be lifted in and out of ambulances, judge each case on its merits.

However, be cautious if in doubt. Many a patient who has just had a myocardial infarction will try to insist there is nothing wrong and want to walk to the ambulance. They must be persuaded not to. A common mistake involves patients who have fainted, because of insufficient blood supply reaching the brain to maintain consciousness, usually due to venous pooling. In this situation the patient needs to be lying flat with feet slightly elevated to improve venous return to the heart and hence cardiac output, which in turn improves blood supply to the brain thereby allowing a regain in consciousness. On occasions emergency personnel arrive to find well-meaning passers-by steadfastly propping the patient upright, and not allowing them to assume a correct horizontal position. Five minutes of lying flat, on oxygen, with legs raised may remove the need for the patient to go to hospital at all.

While relatives and bystanders will no doubt want you to carry the patient to the ambulance, the decision as to whether they walk or not must be made by you, on the basis of their present illness or injury, the effect it is having on them, any underlying conditions and whether walking will worsen their present state. It must be a decision made for medical reasons and in the best interest of the patient but at the same time you do not want to carry patients unncessarily. (It is also worth considering the emotional state of the relatives.)

In the ambulance, consider whether it is best to have the patient sitting or lying in the vehicle and, in what position, how quickly they must be transferred and whether the accident and emergency department need advance warning of your arrival so they can have a doctor and other emergency equipment standing by. Every case, therefore, should be judged individually; but the golden rule must always be to err on the side of caution.

Try to follow up your judgements by enquiring of accident staff how certain patients progressed and what medical diagnosis was finally arrived at. Only in this way can you develop that vital commodity that no textbook can give you, experience. If you got it wrong, this is a positive lesson for the future.

LIFTING TECHNIQUES

The basic principles of lifting are as follows:

(1) Start the lift with legs flexed.
(2) Keep the back straight at all times.
(3) Lift the weight into you, tensing the abdominal muscles.
(4) Straighten the legs as you lift, taking the weight through your legs and off your lower back.

Lifting, however, usually involves two people, so you need to work together as a team, in addition to observing the basic principles outlined above.

The one important difference between solo lifting and two-person lifting is that when two people lift, the weight must be kept as central as possible. If both people lift the weight into themselves then the weakest will end up being pulled forward off balance. Thus more weight must be taken by the arms, and the chair or trolley etc. must be lifted directly upwards. Both crew members can then move into the weight instead of lifting the weight into themselves.

Ambulance crews are rarely matched for height and strength. To lift safely, therefore, you need to work as a pair to the lowest common denominator, that is, the smaller crew member. As people tend to work at different speeds, faster crew members need to slow down a little to accommodate their colleague.

When a crew work together regularly they tend to adapt to each other and find the safest and most effective way of handling situations. However, when two people who do not regularly work together are teamed up, a conscious effort must be made to ensure understanding and teamwork. Check carefully with verbal confirmation, for example, before you lift a patient; if one crew member is very experienced and the other relatively inexperienced, allowances have to made.

Basic Two-person Lifting Technique

The standard technique for lifting a patient is shown in Fig. 16.2.

(1) One person (the taller of the crew members) stands behind the patient, putting his or her arms through the axillae (armpits) of the patient.

(2) The patient's arms are placed across his or her chest, and the taller person grips each arm at the wrist.

(3) The taller person holds the patient's arms close into the chest, ready to lift.

(4) The smaller person crouches to one side of the patient, placing his or her arms under the patient's thighs and small of the back.

(5) They both lift, keeping their backs straight at all times. This will be easier if the taller person is at the patient's head; remember to lift enough to allow the smaller person to stand up straight, avoiding taking any weight on a bent back.

If the patient is to be lifted from the floor the crew member lifting under the legs will be off balance initially and will need to lift the patient up and into him or herself before actually standing up. In this instance the crew member at the head must take most of the weight until their colleague is balanced so that they can both stand up keeping the weight central.

When carrying the patient held in this manner, remember to take small steps only. The crew member at the patient's head can see where they are going much more easily than the other person

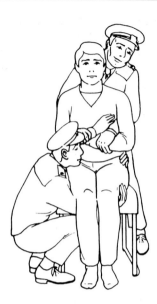

Fig. 16.2   Two-person lifting technique

and may inadvertently take larger strides pulling the other person off balance.

When lifting with a canvas sheet, poles and spreader bars, the principles of straight back, taking the weight on the legs, and a coordinated lift still apply. When transferring the patient, especially if it is over rough ground, both members must walk at the same pace and take small strides to avoid loss of balance.

Use of the Carry Chair

The vast majority of patients are removed from houses using the carry chair. Here again it is better if the taller person takes the top end. Wrap the patient in a blanket and hold the blanket to the chair to secure them, also use the seat belt if available. Tilt the chair back to make lifting and carrying easier but warn the patient that you are going to do this. Patients lifted in a chair may make an involuntary grab at the nearest object as a reflex action if they feel they are going to fall. As that nearest object may be you, a smooth approach to lifting will obviously be to your advantage.

Walking with the chair is most difficult for the person at the bottom as the patient's feet and legs prevent them getting close in to the chair. This person should therefore lead and set the pace. Descend stairs close to the wall, as this offers you a solid object to steady yourself against. Beware hanging pictures and ornaments, however!

Reaching the bottom of a flight of stairs is a particularly dangerous moment as the person at the bottom reaches level ground while the person at the top still has three or four steps to go. It is not uncommon for people to speed up when they reach the foot of the stairs, forgetting that their colleague is still negotiating the steps, thereby pulling them forward; they are then at risk of dropping the patient or falling themselves and possibly injuring their back. Move slowly until your colleague is well and truly on level ground as well. (This also applies when removing the trolley stretcher from the ambulance.)

Use of the Orthopaedic (Scoop) Stretcher

An invaluable aid to moving patients with back injuries, the scoop stretcher (see Appendix B, Fig. B.1b) has the disadvantage that it must be held slightly away from the body when carrying a patient. With a normal stretcher you can stand in between the poles slightly, allowing your arms to be vertical when taking the weight. Carrying a back injury any distance with a scoop can therefore be difficult, and needs a conscious effort to keep your balance and try to hold the stretcher. It is better to use the scoop to lift the patient onto more suitable equipment for transportation. If, however, the scoop stretcher is to be used to carry a patient any distance, you should try to use bystanders to hold the sides of the stretcher as well. This makes it easier to carry and more secure for the patient. Securing straps should be used to keep the patient still.

Use of the Trolley Stretcher

This must be the preferred method of moving a patient as you do not have to take the patient's weight (see Appendix B, Fig. B.2). However, if the ground is rough then the traditional carry stretcher approach is still needed.

Teamwork and understanding in using the trolley stretcher are still essential to avoid the risks of putting excess strain on your colleagues' back or pulling them off balance. The comments made above about lifting at the same time to the same height with straight backs are equally important with this piece of equipment, as are the observations about moving the patient up and down stairs.

When loading the stretcher onto the ambulance, the crew members outside must take care not to go too quickly or they will push their colleague, who is already inside the vehicle, off balance. It may be easier if the first person into the ambulance puts that end of the stretcher down, on the floor, just at the top of the steps rather than trying to carry it all the way into the ambulance. When removing the trolley it is easier to push it out of the ambulance, until only one set of wheels remains on the floor, before the person inside lifts. This means that the person outside the ambulance has to take the weight of their end of the trolley and must pause whilst the person inside lifts before they complete the unloading.

End loading (steps down) or side loading (steps up) is a matter of preference but when side loading care must be taken not to bang the end of the trolley down on the floor of the ambulance. Crews who normally side load may find it safer to end load if the ambulance is on a slope, whereas crews who normally end load may find it much easier to side load with a very heavy patient.

Use of the Paraguard Stretcher

Correct use requires four persons, which makes coordination of the move that much more difficult. A clear plan of action in advance is necessary if all are to work together to keep the paraguard stable and under control. This is particularly true in confined spaces and both crews must work together with one person giving the instructions.

POSITIONING THE PATIENT ON THE STRETCHER

There are nine positions as follows.

Recumbent

As Fig. 16.3 shows, patients lie flat on their backs with one pillow supporting the head. This is most suitable for back or pelvic injuries, suspected fractures of the hip or femur, or any

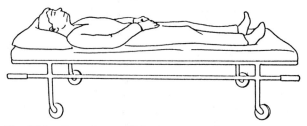

Fig. 16.3   Stretcher positioning: recumbent or supine

condition where the patient feels dizzy or lightheaded sitting up-right. This also includes heart attacks with a bradycardia or any arrhythmia which is causing a low blood pressure (e.g. atrial fibrillation, ventricular tachycardia) and is now the preferred position for gynaecological haemorrhage (but check with your local maternity unit to ensure they do not still want the legs raised). Check the patient's breathing as this position may cause problems, especially in the elderly. It may also cause a patient to feel nauseous.

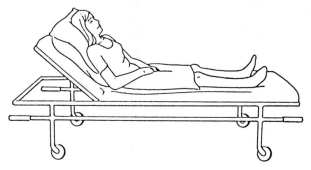

Fig. 16.4   Stretcher positioning: semi-recumbent

Semi-recumbent

The majority of patients for whom there is no special contraindi-cation will find this the most comfortable position (Fig. 16.4).

Semi-recumbent Half-turned

This position is of use for a person who has suffered trauma to one side of the chest. Have the injured side down (the right side in Fig. 16.5) so the patient may make maximum use of the unin-jured lung.

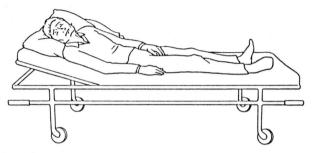

Fig. 16.5   Stretcher positioning: semi-recumbent, half-turned

Upright

As Fig. 16.6a shows, the patient is as near 90° as possible, the

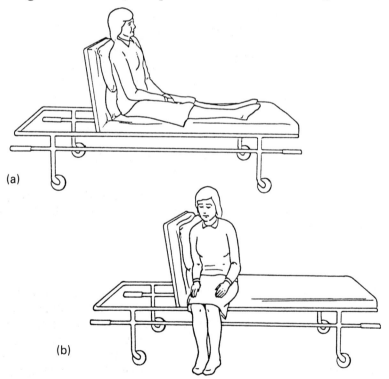

(a)

(b)

Fig. 16.6   Stretcher positioning, upright: (a) with legs on the stretcher;
(b) with legs down

best position for someone with breathing difficulties. If patients wish to sit on the trolley with their legs hanging over the side they should be allowed to do so (Fig. 16.6b). This is especially important in cardiac conditions such as acute congestive heart failure or left ventricular failure. It will help the breathing difficulties by reducing pulmonary oedema. *Note:* where breathing difficulties are caused by chest conditions or pulmonary oedema the patient will want to sit up. Listen to them.

Fowler's

From Fig. 16.7 we can see that this position allows patients to relax their abdominal muscles. It is therefore recommended for acute abdominal emergencies and injuries. Patients who have

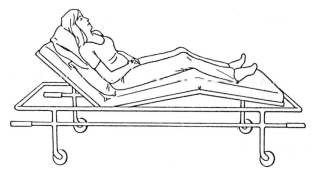

Fig. 16.7   Stretcher positioning: Fowler's

suffered heart attacks and who are being moved in the semi-recumbent position sometimes find it more comfortable if their legs are raised in this manner.

Legs Raised

To achieve this position, as shown in Fig. 16.8a tilt the top part of the stretcher head down, then raise the top half into a horizontal plane. This position will improve venous return to the heart and therefore circulation in the vital heart/lung system, making it the position of choice in dealing with shocked patients. The patient is not positioned head down because although this will not dramatically affect arterial blood supply to the brain (autonomically controlled) it will affect venous return from the brain

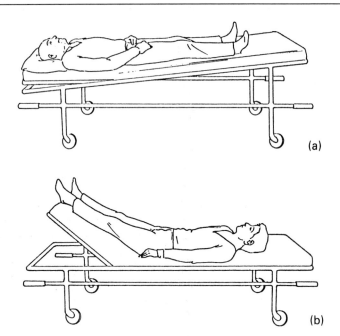

Fig. 16.8   Stretcher positioning: (a) legs raised: (b) high elevation of legs

(gravity controlled) thus causing congestion in the cerebral blood vessels and a possible increase in intercranial pressure.

If the patients' blood pressures are unrecordable or very low (systolic below 75), or their condition indicates major blood loss, they may be laid with their feet at the head end (Fig. 16.8b), which allows for even greater elevation. This can also be used in severe anaphylactic shock.

Positioning the Unconscious Patient

We have already discussed the threat to the unconscious person's airway (see p. 3) and some of the steps that may help keep it clear. It is essential that everything be done in transit to keep this airway clear, and the correct way to achieve this is with the recovery position shown in Fig. 16.9.

Patients are placed on their side, lower leg straight, upper leg bent at 90°, lower arm behind their back, top arm in front of the face. Remember to have the neck extended to keep the tongue clear of the airway. A coma roll blanket will be of assistance;

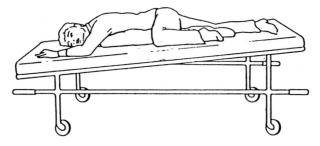

Fig. 16.9   Stretcher positioning: recovery

spread it out lengthways, bring the bottom end two-thirds of the way to the top then roll the blanket across. The thick end supports the chest and abdomen while the thin end supports the top leg. If vomiting occurs, the bottom of the trolley should be raised to facilitate drainage from the mouth. This head down position should only be maintained for the minimum period of time due to its possible adverse effects on intracranial pressure.

Prone

This is most useful in dealing with the patient who has severe facial injuries as it allows easy drainage of blood, thereby avoiding the threat to the airway or the risk of blood being swallowed which will in turn lead to vomiting (Fig. 16.10).

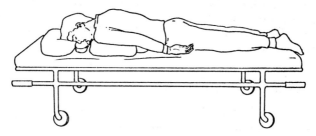

Fig. 16.10   Stretcher positioning: prone

Knee–Elbow

This position (Fig. 16.11) is for use with a pregnant woman in labour who has a prolapsed cord (see Chapter 8, p. 130).

Due to the nature of the patient's injuries or general condition it may not always be possible to adopt the positions suggested above. Compromise is sometimes needed. However, never lose sight of the basic principles of what you are trying to do, whether it be to keep an airway clear, assist breathing, or improve venous return in a shocked patient, and you should then be able to work out the best position.

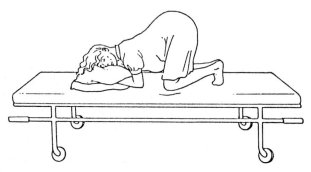

Fig. 16.11   Stretcher positioning: prone, knee–elbow

Whatever position is adopted, ensure that the patient is well wrapped up with blankets. They give a feeling of comfort and in winter are essential to keep the patient warm, especially if they are only wearing night attire.

Remember also to keep a white carrying canvas on the stretcher, under the blanket, so that poles can be used to move the patient, at their destination, if necessary. Keep an inconti-pad opened out between the canvas and the blanket (in the middle) so that if a patient unexpectedly fouls the blanket it will not go through to the canvas.

SCOOP AND RUN OR STAY AND STABILISE?

This question has aroused much fierce debate over the years. It reflects two opposing schools of thought about the best way to manage an injured or seriously ill patient in the field.

Over the last decade or so, great strides have been made in ambulance service training with the result that treatment can now be given in the field that will stabilise a patient's condition and greatly assist the chances of recovery. Members of the public, however, still expect that an ambulance will automatically 'rush the patient to hospital', a phrase beloved of the media and used a great deal in describing accidents.

Sometimes you may find your efforts at preserving life, preventing further deterioration in the patient's condition and promoting recovery are interpreted by irate members of the public as wasting time. They *want* the patient rushed to hospital for treatment.

Ambulance personnel are moving on from the position of learning treatments for conditions parrot fashion. The demands of the 1980s and 90s require substantial theoretical knowledge. We need the ability to recognise conditions and the dangers associated with them, the ability to decide upon priorities and treatments, and most of all the practical skills to carry out those treatments. The decision of whether to treat first and move later, or move first and try to treat en route, can only be made correctly with the benefit of this knowledge and practical capability.

With the advent of extended training, ambulance personnel are now able to bring the kind of immediate care to the patient which at one time was only available in hospitals. Bear in mind though that both the patient and the relatives may not understand this. They must be given an explanation of the treatment you are giving and of the benefit it will bring to the patient. This of course applies to any ambulance aid given. We must never forget the value of reassurance. It is an essential part of good patient care.

If the patient is going to be rushed to an accident and emergency unit, consideration should be given to the effect a very fast and uncomfortable ride may have, together with flashing blue lights and sirens. Would you believe the attendant who was telling you that you were going to be fine and that there was nothing to worry about? Chapter 11 showed how patients take emotional cues from the people and situation around them, hence the need for emergency personnel to be calm and reassuring in their manner. Think very carefully of the disadvantages that such a journey may have before embarking upon it. Are the few minutes you might gain worth it?

One example will illustrate how things may go horribly wrong with the rush to hospital approach. A voluntary ambulance was covering a large event, a person collapsed with cardiac arrest, panic ensued which resulted in the unfortunate person being bundled into the back of the ambulance while a volunteer officer of the organisation ordered the young and inexperienced driver to get to hospital as fast as possible. This he proceeded to do, but in such a wildly erratic way that there was nothing the attendant in the back of the vehicle could do for the patient. The result was that the patient's airway was full of vomit, he had had no oxygen or cardiac massage, and was beyond any medical help when they arrived at the accident and emergency department.

Among the many morals of this sad tale is the fact that if you are going to move a patient quickly, it must be done at a speed that allows the attendant actually to treat the patient in the back of the vehicle. The moral about not panicking is plain to see, as is the fact that you can try to work *too* fast. Your optimum speed is that which still allows you to treat the patient effectively. To try to work faster is counterproductive.

It is worth considering also the effect a dramatic arrival has on the accident and emergency staff, who will assume you have a serious emergency on board. If you have not, however, your credibility and that of your colleagues and the service in general will suffer. Accident and emergency staff do take note of ambulance crew, and their opinions will determine how much attention they pay to you and the information you bring with you about the patient in the future. That is only human nature. For the sake of a good working relationship, therefore, think carefully about how much drama needs to be attached to your arrival!

Advantages of a Stay and Stabilise Policy

These can be summarised as follows.

(1) It allows a thorough assessment to be made, so the patient's problems and general condition can be more reliably determined.
(2) There are great psychological benefits for the patient, if rushing and stress can be avoided.
(3) Treatment of major problems can begin at once, such as correct airway management or an intravenous infusion for shock, and can be continued en route.
(4) Improvement or deterioration in the patient's condition can be monitored en route and the hospital informed on arrival.

(5) Accident and emergency staff will take you seriously when you do arrive with sirens and blue lights.

If Urgent Transfer to Hospital is Necessary

At the same time it must be remembered that there will be occasions when remaining at the scene may be detrimental to the patient. How do you decide? Use the following criteria:

(1) How close is the hospital?
(2) Have you been able to fully diagnose and assess the condition of the patient?
(3) Are you able to treat the patient's acute needs at the scene in the ambulance and to stabilise their condition?
(4) Are they responding to your treatment?
(5) Are there any over-riding circumstances, such as riot conditions or traumatic amputations (where urgent surgical intervention may save a limb), which necessitate moving immediately.

Each situation must be assessed on its merits. No matter how serious it is, there must be some sort of assessment before deciding on rational action. If the decision is to go to hospital as a matter of urgency, the golden rule to remember is that speed must be *effective*. In other words you must travel quickly to save time, but not too quickly that the attendant cannot manage the patient en route. The ride should be fast but smooth and controlled. The driver should not give way to the emotion of the situation; use headlights and flashing lights by all means, but use of sirens should be kept to a minimum due to the adverse effect this may have on the patient's stress levels, particularly in shock related conditions.

With the benefit of sound theoretical knowledge and learning from experience, emergency personnel should be able to make a rational decision based on their assessment of what needs doing on scene and how quickly the journey to hospital needs to be made. If in doubt erring on the side of caution is of course the final piece of guidance. Careful consideration of each case with appropriate action taken in the field is a better policy than 'scoop and run regardless'!

17. Legal Aspects of Ambulance Work

INTRODUCTION

Apart from driving exemptions, the law does not convey any legal powers on ambulance personnel beyond that of the ordinary citizen. Thus if people are forced into an ambulance and taken to hospital against their will, or their home is broken into by ambulance personnel because a neighbour fears they might be ill, they may proceed against the ambulance personnel in law. Obviously this would mean them suing the health authority because you are acting as their agent but your actions would be closely scrutinised and after the court case you may also be called upon to answer for them by your own service.

USING FORCE, AND THE
MENTAL HEALTH ACT

If the person who was forcibly removed to hospital was under an appropriate section of the Mental Health Act, the ambulance crew will have a defence in law. If the ambulance crew broke into the person's house because they genuinely believed that person would come to harm otherwise, they will have a defence. What can be seen therefore is that while the law does not convey rights on ambulance personnel, it does allow a defence for actions taken, provided those acts were believed to be in the patient's best interests.

One further ingredient the law requires of ambulance personnel is that where they are called upon to use force, only a reasonable amount to accomplish the task in hand may be used. Thus if you put your arms around a patient who is sectioned under the Mental Health Act, to restrain them, this would be said to be a reasonable amount of force, but if you then hit them to keep them quiet this would be a wilful act. The principle of reasonable force applies also to self-defence if a crew member is attacked by a patient. Every citizen has a right to self-defence but only within these limitations.

REFUSAL TO GO TO HOSPITAL

Ambulance crew will often encounter the difficult situation of patients they feel ought to go to hospital but who refuse; or perhaps friends or relatives are adamant that they must go. If they are forced aboard a vehicle, they may consequently sue for common assault as ambulance personnel have *no legal right* to take people anywhere against their wishes.

In the case of a patient with mental problems, therefore, before you use force you must ensure that they have been sectioned and are not just a voluntary admission. The mental welfare officer or a doctor should be at the scene to show you the papers and if not (but Control informs you that the patient is sectioned) you are quite within your rights to ask the relatives to give you written permission to use force. Remember that even reasonable force should be applied as tactfully as possible.

Where the Mental Health Act is not in force you cannot remove patients against their will. The best thing to do if they refuse to come with you, therefore, is to contact their GP, if the patient is at home, or the police if they are not. Do not leave the scene until they arrive if you feel that the patient is in danger, but do not take it upon yourself to remove the patient by force.

PRIVATE PROPERTY

A similar argument applies to the question of breaking into patients' private property. Unless you are absolutely sure that the person is in there and is in imminent danger do not break in yourself but ask Control to contact the police to get them to the scene to gain entry. If you decide that you must gain entry yourself then try only to cause the minimum amount of damage necessary to do so. Here again the property owner may seek redress for the damage done. If a property has been broken into, the police must be informed in order that it may be secured. Failure to do this may lead to the property being burgled, and the ambulance crew responsible being sued for damages. If it is necessary to leave before the police arrive, it is important to try to find a volunteer who will be responsible for the property until the police are present. The name and address should be noted and passed on to Control where it may be correctly recorded.

PERSONAL PROPERTY

A common problem involves patient's property such as handbags, shopping, spectacles, etc. that may accidentally get lost in transit to hospital. Ambulance personnel are responsible for the safekeeping of a patient's personal effects, and the patient is entitled to seek legal redress if items disappear. So if possible ensure that the patient's property is taken into the A&E department with the patient and not left unattended on the ambulance outside. If on moving a patient you are asked to sign for their property, check it and ensure that on your log sheet you also get a signature for the property from the person receiving the patient. In addition to taking care of property in transit to hospital, ensure that hospital staff are made fully aware of the patient's property; it should not just be left by the trolley in the patient's cubicle on the premise that accident and emergency nursing staff will guess it belongs to the patient.

Property accidentally left on the ambulance is the crew's responsibility until handed over to an ambulance officer or the police. Property found at the scene of an accident should be handed over to the police for safekeeping. It cannot be overemphasised how much care should be taken over patients' property as it is the source of many complaints both in hospital and in the field. A great deal of unpleasantness is associated with allegations of theft which the police have to investigate thoroughly.

It is a sobering thought, but any experienced accident and emergency nurse will readily describe admitting elderly patients who often look poorly dressed, yet turn out to have thousands of pounds concealed about their person. Great care must therefore be taken with patients' effects; the alternative is a complaint that will have to be thoroughly investigated by senior officers and possibly the police, and may end up in court. Either criminal or civilian proceedings are possible, and the result will be a long drawn-out and worrying time for the ambulance personnel involved.

SUDDEN OR UNNATURAL DEATH

By the nature of ambulance work, crew will often be involved in cases of sudden, violent or unnatural death. All cases must be reported to the coroner and there will need to be a post-mortem unless the patient's GP (or hospital doctor if they died in hospital) is prepared to sign a death certificate stating the cause of death. The doctor can only do this if he or she has seen the patient within the last fourteen days and was treating the patient for the condition which caused the death. Other than this, the doctor can only pronounce death and a post-mortem must be held to establish the cause.

On arrival at a scene where a person is beyond any resuscitation attempt, the correct step is to notify the police immediately and await them. The police are the coroner's representatives and the body *may not be moved* until they give permission. The other legal requirement is for a doctor formally to pronounce death; this may be the family doctor, or if the death has occurred in a public place, a casualty officer at the nearest accident and emergency unit.

If deceased are in their own home, there is no need for the ambulance crew to remove the body. This will be done either by the family making their own funeral arrangements if the general practitioner is prepared to certify death, or the police or duty funeral director taking over responsibility for the body. If the body is not in the deceased's home, it must be removed to the accident and emergency unit for a doctor to pronounce death and then on to the mortuary. Local policy will vary around these basic principles. So it is important that personnel are fully aware of this and observe the rules very carefully.

In the case of suspicious circumstances surrounding a person's death, the police should be called immediately and the suspicious circumstances stressed. This will ensure a rapid police response. If resuscitation is attempted every effort should be made to disturb things as little as possible although in reality this may not be very feasible. The police should also be notified quickly if resuscitation is attempted on a person suffering serious injuries associated with suspicious circumstances. Gunshot wounds are *automatically* notifiable to the police whatever their severity.

Ambulance crew who find a body must stay with the body until it is handed over to the police. If there is a subsequent murder trial, the prosecution have to account for the safekeeping of the body from discovery to post-mortem in order that there may be no suspicion of tampering with it. It might be very damaging to the prosecution's case if it is discovered that the ambulance crew summoned to the scene left the body unattended for any period of time.

DYING DECLARATIONS

Seriously injured patients may give the ambulance crew vital information about how their injuries were sustained. If they believe they are dying and subsequently do die, this is known as a 'dying declaration' and is admissible in court as evidence if a person is subsequently charged with murder or manslaughter. The judge needs to be satisfied that the deceased was dying and aware of it at the time, that the deceased knew there was no hope of recovery, and that the statement relates to the cause of death. This is *crucial testimony*, so if ambulance personnel find themselves in this situation, they should write down what is said as soon as possible and give that information to the police.

Emergency personnel need to be fully aware of the potential legal problems involved in their work. Careful adherence to local procedures and policy is therefore strongly recommended for your own protection and peace of mind.

Appendix A

Transport of Hazardous Goods— United Kingdom Hazard Information System

HAZCHEM CARD

This must be displayed by all road tankers carrying hazardous goods. It should be located on both sides of the vehicle and at the rear and measure 40×70 cm (Fig. A.1).

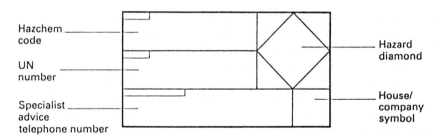

Hazchem code

UN number

Specialist advice telephone number

Hazard diamond

House/ company symbol

Fig. A.1   The Hazchem card

Hazchem Code

The Hazchem code identifies the action to be taken by the fire brigade. It is a combination of a number (indicating which fire-fighting agent to use) and a letter which indicates the breathing apparatus required. If the code is followed by the letter E, this indicates the need for evacuation of all non-essential personnel from the immediate area.

United Nations (UN) Number

The United Nations (UN) number is an internationally recognised labelling system that identifies the substance on board. This number should be given to Control by any vehicle at the scene. If more than one substance is carried, the UN code number will be replaced by the word 'Multiload'. Each tanker compartment will then have the UN number displayed on its side.

Hazard Warning Diamond

Each hazard-warning diamond relates to a group of substances and describes the danger that group poses—for example, poison, pressurised gas. The presence of an exclamation mark indicates more than one hazard.

Telephone Number

The specialist advice telephone number given on the Hazchem sign should be manned when the vehicle is mobile. If the sign states 'Contact Local Depot' the name of the company should be on the side of the tanker. Control will need this number.

EUROPEAN ROAD TRANSPORT SYSTEM, KEMIER CODE

The Kemier code should be displayed by all tankers carrying hazardous substances to and from Europe. The sign is 40×30 cm and should be displayed on both sides and at the front of the vehicle (Fig. A.2).

The Kemier code consists of two or three digits. The first digit indicates the primary hazard involved, while secondary or tertiary hazards are given by the subsequent digits (Table A.1). If the same digit is repeated, this indicates intensification of the

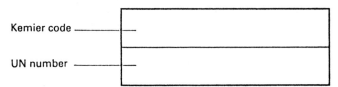

Fig. A.2   The Kemier code

hazard. An X in front of a number means do not bring in contact with water. The UN number is displayed as in the Hazchem system.

Table A.1 Kemier Code Digits

First digit	Second/third digit
2 Gas	0 No meaning
3 Inflammable liquid	1 Explosion risk
4 Inflammable solid	2 Gas may be given off
5 Oxidising substance or organic peroxide	3 Inflammable risk
	5 Oxidising risk
6 Toxic substance	6 Toxic risk
7 Radioactive material	8 Corrosive risk
8 Corrosive	9 Violent reaction risk

RADIOACTIVE MATERIALS

The distinctive international symbol denoting the presence of radioactivity is shown in Fig. A.3. It should be displayed on all vehicles transporting radioactive materials—and on any building where they are stored.

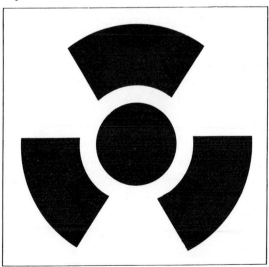

Fig. A.3   The international symbol for radioactivity, in practice the symbol is displayed on a yellow background

Appendix B
Ambulance Equipment – Basic and Extended

BASIC

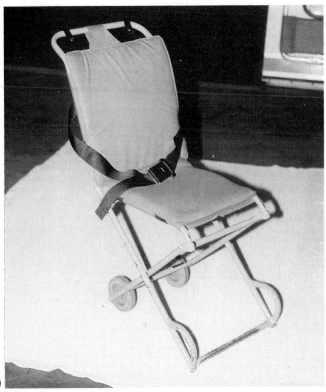

(a)

Fig. B.1(a) Basic ambulance carry chair (collapsible). Some varieties have four wheels. Note the seat belt, which should always be used with a patient on the chair. It secures the patient and allows you to take a firm, unencumbered grip on the chair

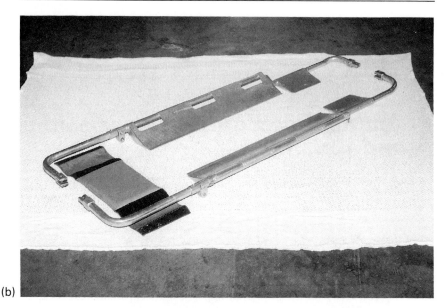

(b)

Fig. B.1(b) Orthopaedic (scoop) stretcher. Its main use is in picking up a patient without altering his or her position, such as in back injury, but it can be extremely useful in other situations, for example, moving a patient from bed with several drips *in situ*. The stretcher should be measured against the patient and altered in length before being parted. *Caution*: The pillow's velcrose fittings can sometimes pull apart when lifting. To avoid this the hands at the top should be placed so that the fingers can hold the pillow flaps, as well as the bars, as the stretcher is lifted. Straps can be obtained so that the patient can be strapped to the stretcher if necessary. The head end should be closed first when placing under the patient. The foot end should be opened first when removing from under the patient. Watch that the patient's clothes do not catch in the middle as the stretcher is closed. *Note*: The pillow is positioned to show the velcrose which should be placed on top of the bars and fastened underneath

Opposite:
Fig. B.2 York 4 trolley stretcher. This shows the stretcher in the elevated position, back raised, base of the stretcher in the Fowler position (see Fig. 16.7) (by turning the black knob on the right-hand side) and with the bottom end elevated in the drainage position (handle is on the right-hand side)

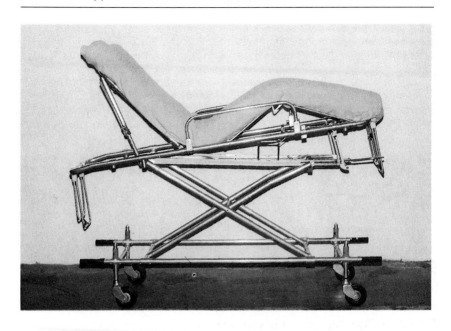

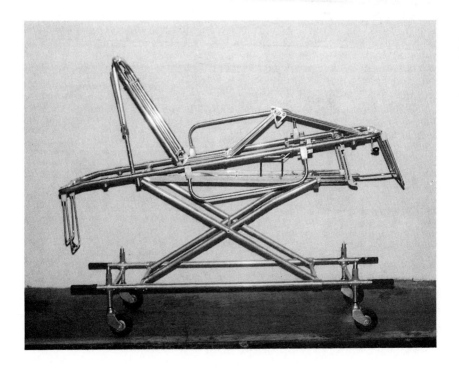

Fig. B.3(a) Fracpac—immobiliser splint. This forms a box splint around a damaged limb. One padding should be placed under the leg in the splint; the other can either be placed on top of the leg to complete the box, or be used as a 'U'-shaped padding around the foot to give extra support to a lower leg injury. The black straps are then fastened across to prevent movement. A long wooden splint is available which fits inside one side of the Fracpac to provide a long leg splint for a fractured hip. Fracstraps are also available to secure the splint and the Fracpac to the body and the other leg

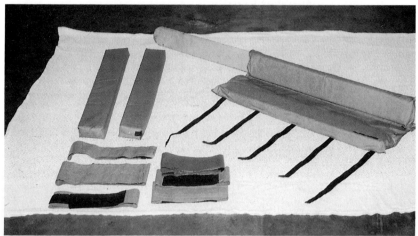

(a)

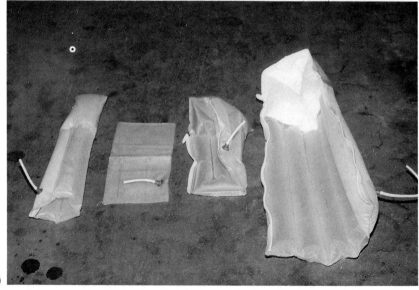

(b)

Fig. B.3(b) Inflatable splints. The splint is placed around the limb and zipped up before inflating. They should be blown up by mouth to avoid overinflation. The white tube is pulled out to open the valve and pushed in to close it. They are useful in a simple straight fracture and also to apply direct pressure over a bleeding wound, but it must be borne in mind that the splint applies an overall pressure and it may, therefore, straighten a deformed limb irrespective of the damage caused. Overinflation may also result in interference with the circulation and it may push protruding bones back into the limb, so it should be used with caution. The splints come in four sizes: long arm, short arm, long leg, short leg

Fig. B.4 Wooden spinal board (front view). This is for removing a patient with a whiplash or spinal injury from a car or lorry etc. A cervical collar is fitted to the patient. The board is then slid down behind the patient and a skull bandage is used to secure the head against the pad on the board. Padding is placed behind the head and neck, if necessary, to avoid overextension, and the ends of the bandage tied into whichever indent is correct for height. The upper straps are placed as shown (not through the hand holds) and the lower straps go down the inside of the groin, up the outside of the leg and across the front of the body to join the opposite upper strap (ensure that they are tight). The knees and feet are tied together and the patient is removed and placed on the stretcher in that position with the legs supported. The straps are released and the legs are gently lowered to the stretcher. If patients are unconscious, they can be placed on their side on the stretcher and the lower leg can either be released, to give a semirecovery position, or left tied and strapped depending on their other injuries

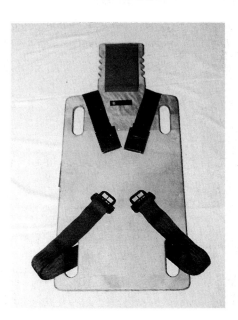

Fig. B.5 KED extrication device (rear view). This device is mainly used to remove spinal injuries from cars or lorries etc. but can be used for a fractured hip or pelvis. It is very flexible and is easy to apply and use. The steps are basically the same as for the wooden board but padding is supplied for the neck and head (bottom of picture). Chin and head pads are also supplied (middle of picture) which fasten to the side of the head supports. (The chin support must be removed if the patient vomits.) The chest straps are done up first followed by the leg straps, which are placed under the leg on the same side, up through the groin and then fastened to the opposite side of the KED (the ends of the straps are colour coded). The head is then secured to the support. While fitting the KED ensure that the top of the chest section is right up under the armpits. The patient can then be removed and placed on the stretcher as previously stated. At this point the patient's airway and breathing must be checked to ensure that the chin strap (which may now be removed) and the chest straps are not too tight or causing interference. *Note*: The top chest strap is the final thing to be done up, just prior to removing the patient, and it should be loosened once the patient is on the stretcher. (See the Ferno KED training poster for a fuller explanation)

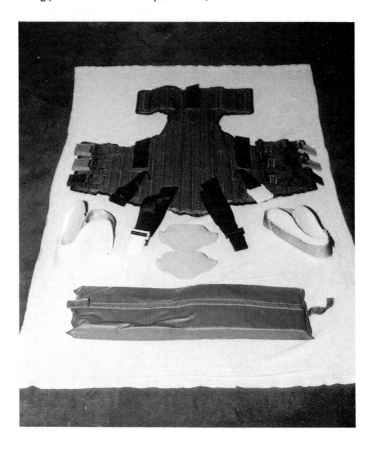

Fig. B.6 Entonox equipment. Entonox is an analgesic gas which contains 50% oxygen and 50% nitrous oxide. Note that the gases will separate at temperatures below approximately −7°C. The gas comes in a blue cylinder with white quarters on the shoulders. A 'D' size cylinder is carried on an ambulance. It must be held by the patient and self-administered except in exceptional circumstances, such as two broken arms. The equipment contains a demand valve which means the patient must suck in the gas to make it work. This causes a noise; listen for this noise to ensure the patient is breathing in Entonox and not rebreathing his or her own expired air. Ensure that the mask is tight against the face to form a seal. *Never leave a patient on Entonox alone.* They may relax completely with the mask over their face, thus rebreathing their own expired air, and possibly asphyxiate. Entonox may cause funny effects—for example, patients may feel as if they are floating away or get pins and needles. This must be explained to them when they are told how to use the gas, or they may become frightened and refuse to use it. The gas enters the blood stream via the lungs and leaves the body the same way when the patient stops using it. When not in use, the key to turn the cylinder on should be placed in the exit tube to keep out dust.

Entonox should not be given to: Patients who are drunk (airway danger). Mental patients (the patient must understand what they are doing). Head injuries with impaired consciousness (airway danger). Divers with the bends (will exacerbate the condition). Maxillofacial injuries (probably unable to use; airway danger). Unconscious patients or those who refuse. Chest injuries with a risk of a pneumothorax (will exacerbate the condition)

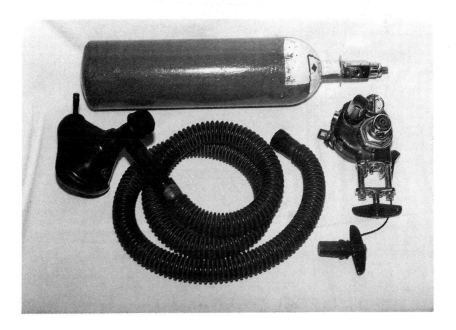

Fig. B7 Suction equipment. The example shown here is the *Laerdal Aspirator* (rechargeable from the vehicle batteries). The pump is seen on the left of the aspirator (including the pump bottle). The central container is for aspirated contents, and the small bottle on the right-hand side should contain water so that it can be sucked up into the tube if it blocks with vomit. This model contains its own batteries so that it can be used away from the vehicle. There are a number of different types of aspirator available and whichever one you have you should make sure that you know how to use it
Suction catheters (laid out below the Laerdal Aspirator). Types shown are: *Yankaur* (top). This is for clearing the upper airway and throat. The hole in the upper part of the catheter must be blocked with the finger to cause suction up through the tube. Put the sucker into the mouth, block the hole and withdraw slowly at the same time to suck out contents. *Endotracheal*: large-bore (middle), small-bore (bottom). This is used through an endotracheal tube (ET) to clear the trachea and lungs of fluid. It can also be used to clear the nasal passages of a patient, especially one who is fitting and only breathing through the nose. When inserting pinch the tube between the fingers, to prevent suction, and then release it and withdraw slowly, at the same time, to remove contents

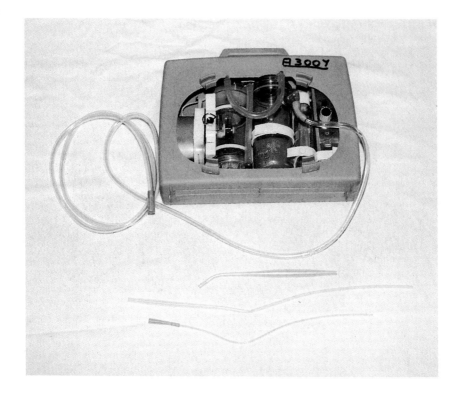

Fig. B.8 Resuscitation bags. Paediatric and adult Ambu bag is on the right. Laerdal adult and child bag on the left. (This contains a valve in the neck which, when released, allows excess air or air and oxygen to exhaust into the air.) All the bags shown have an inlet tube to which an oxygen supply can be attached which will give a mixture of air and oxygen (6 litres/min in an adult bag will give approximately 50% mixture; turn the supply down slightly if the bag begins to over inflate). To achieve a 100% oxygen supply a reservoir or a cap (adult Ambu bag) must be attached. Ensure that all the valves are *in situ* and are working before using the bags. The bags will attach directly to an endotracheal tube but a connector should be used if possible (see Fig. B.9)

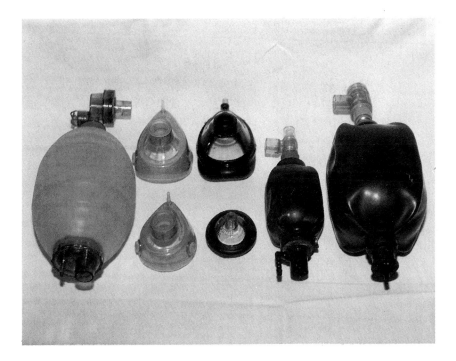

EXTENDED

Fig. B.9 Intubation equipment. *Magills forceps* (top). This is for removing debris from the mouth and throat and for nasal intubations. *Intubation tubes* (various sizes). Smaller tubes do not have cuffs. Intubate until the tube stops as indicated by the black line. There are two types of cuff on the larger tubes (Portex): (1) low volume, high pressure cuff; (2) high volume, low pressure cuff. The first may be found slightly easier to use due to the size of the cuff. *Small artery forceps*. These are used for sealing the neck of the cuff inflation tube (above the sight bag). The sight bag shows if the cuff is inflated and will begin to deflate if the cuff is leaking. *Intubation tube (cuff inflated), connection and Laerdal resuscitation bag*. A connection should always be used between the intubation tube and the resuscitation bag if possible. Its flexibility helps to avoid the tube being moved by the bag, as ventilation is carried out, and endotracheal suction can be performed by removing the cap over the top of the connector, directly over the top of the tube (always ensure that the cap is in place when ventilating). *Syringe 20 ml*. This is used for inflating the cuff. Inflate lungs and squeeze syringe (at the same time) until the noise of air passing the tube stops. Do not overinflate the cuff as it may cause trachea damage. *Laryngoscopes* (paediatric and adult). Always carry spare bulbs and batteries. Having intubated, always check that both lungs are inflating evenly and that the tube is tied in securely

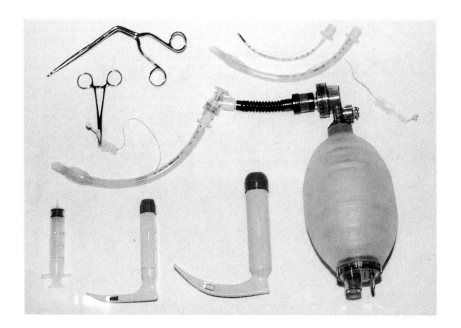

Fig. B.10 Infusion equipment. *Infusion fluids*. Fluids shown (left to right) are: Hartmann's; 0.9% sodium chloride (normal saline); 5% dextrose; Haemaccel. Always check the following before using: (1) The correct fluid is being used. (2) The fluid is in date. (3) The outer bag is intact and no fluid can be seen between the two bags; take off the outer bag. (4) The fluid in the inner bag is clear, not discoloured and contains no particulate matter (invert the bag several times). *Giving set*. Check that the wrapper is intact, the set is in date and the ends of the giving set are still covered before using. Set up the infusion as follows: (1) Twist the end off the giving set (filter end) and insert into the bag. (2) Ensure that the roller is switched off and hang the bag up. (3) Fill up the filter chamber (top) (pinch the pump chamber (bottom) while doing so). Then half fill the pump chamber. (4) Open the roller fully and hold the other end lower than the chambers. The fluid will run through to the end. Check there are no air bubbles in the tube. Close the roller, remove the cover and insert the end into the venflon. Twist the end to secure (Leur lock fitting). (5) Open the roller fully for a few seconds, allowing the fluid to flow, and then set to required flow rate (aseptic technique). Sometimes the fluid does not flow freely in someone whose blood pressure is low, or if the end of the venflon is against a valve in the vein. To push the fluid through, fill *both* chambers and either gently squeeze the pump chamber or, if a fast infusion is necessary, squeeze the bag. Once the infusion is running freely, shut off the roller, invert the bag and pump some of the fluid from the chambers back into

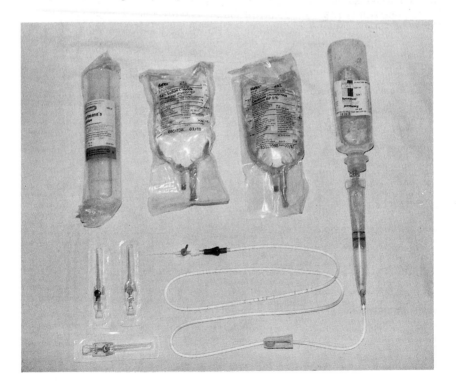

the bag. Then reset the chambers so that you can watch how the infusion is running and restart it. *Venflons.* Once a venflon is successfully inserted the blood in the tube must be prevented from clotting. This is achieved by either setting up a slow running drip, or by flushing it through with, for example, 5 ml of Hepsal. The time of starting the drip or of flushing it through must be recorded for the hospital. Always check the end of the venflon, in the vein, for tissuing, on commencement of a drip or when flushing it through. A sizeable bubble will appear, under the skin, very quickly (immediately if flushing) if the venflon is not in the vein. Tape the venflon securely or bandage the arm to a short arm splint before moving the patient. Aseptic techniques should be used when inserting a venflon and the skin above the vein should be cleaned with a Steret prior to insertion. Venflons are colour coded according to gauge as follows: blue—22 gauge; pink—20 gauge; green—18 gauge; yellow—17 gauge; grey—16 gauge; brown—14 gauge (brown is the largest)

Fig. B.11 Cardiac monitor and defibrillator. Example shown here is the Lifepak 5, which is a separate ECG monitor and defibrillator joined together. The batteries are interchangeable. It has the ability to: (1) monitor the patient, via a three-lead ECG, shown visually on the cardioscope; (2) provide a printed readout of the ECG; (3) monitor through the defibrillator paddles which is also shown visually on the cardioscope; (4) defibrillate the patient—by using an unsynchronised shock (ventricular fibrillation); (5) provide cardioversion, in the case of ventricular tachycardia, by using a synchronised shock. *Always remember the following*: (1) The most important thing to consider, when monitoring a patient, is the patient's condition and the effect any arrhythmia

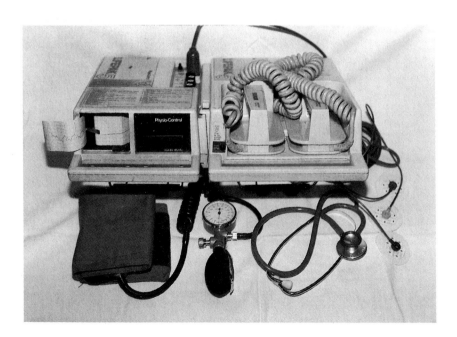

is having on him or her, not the arrhythmia itself. (2) Patient details, plus pulse and blood pressure, should always be written on every printed readout; the time and date of the ECG should also be shown. (3) When defibrillating a patient always ensure everyone is clear of the patient; watch for people leaning against a metal bed or trolley without realising it. (4) A manual is provided with every type of ECG monitor and/or defibrillator. You should always ensure you have read the manual thoroughly before using the machine. *Never* rely on other people explaining it to you

Fig. B.12 Drugs and miscellaneous. All the drugs shown are in prepacked syringes from International Medication Systems (UK) Ltd of Daventry. The ends of the syringes are colour-coded, for ease of application, and the two parts simply screw together. Methylprednisolone contains three containers because the powder needs to be mixed with the diluent before being assembled. (a). Methylprednisolone 500 mg, a steroid for reducing cerebral oedema. (b) Atropine sulphate 1 mg in 10 ml, for use in bradycardia and asystole. (c) Lignocaine 1% 100 mg in 10 ml, for use in ventricular tachycardia, multiventricular ectopics and coarse ventricular fibrillation which will not revert. (d) Adrenaline 1:10 000, 10 ml, for use in asystole and fine ventricular fibrillation which will not revert. (e) Sodium bicarbonate 8.4% 50 ml, used to reverse metabolic acidosis. (f) Dextrose 50% 50 ml, used to reverse a hypoglycaemic diabetic coma. Atropine, lignocaine and adrenaline can be given either intravenously or via the endotracheal tube; methylprednisolone, sodium bicarbonate and dextrose must be given intravenously. *Miscellaneous. Needles*: 23 gauge (blue end) can be used for

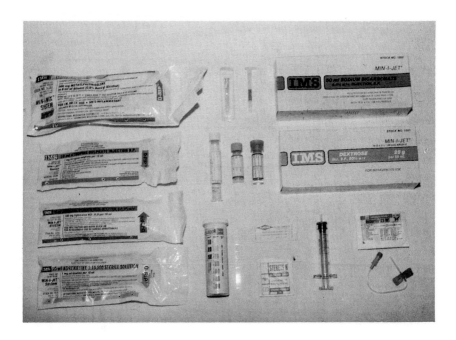

obtaining blood for a BM stick test; 21 gauge (green end) used for drawing up Hepsal etc. *Blood sample bottles*: general bottle (no anticoagulant) 10 ml, bottle with white top; fluoride oxalate 2.5 ml, bottle with yellow top; EDTA 4 ml, bottle with lilac top. *BM sticks*: average normal reading is 5.5 on the scale; cover both parts with blood and always wipe stick sideways. *Lancets*: used for obtaining blood for a BM stick test. *Sterets*: used for cleaning a site prior to inserting a venflon etc. *Syringes*: 5 ml, for drawing up Hepsal; 20 ml, for taking blood for blood samples, and intubation (inflating cuff). *Butterfly*: 19, 21 gauge, useful for drugs or even dextrose in a hypoglycaemic diabetic with no visible veins. *Hepsal*: 5 ml phials, used for flushing through venflons and butterflies to prevent blood, or fluid clotting or solidifying in them

Fig. B.13 Oxygen Resuscitators. (a) *Sabre Saturn*. Delivers oxygen and air to a set *pressure*. The amount of oxygen delivered can be increased by blocking the air inlet with your finger, but this interferes with the cycle and it must be removed each time to allow the lungs to exhaust their contents. (b) *Pneu PAC*. Delivers 100% oxygen to a set *volume*. Both use a 'D' size oxygen cylinder (black with all-white shoulders and neck). Both can be used for resuscitation purposes or for oxygen therapy (tubing and fitments are supplied). Both have a means of adjusting the amount delivered according to the patient's size. Both have a contents gauge: Sabre Saturn has a normal glass gauge. In the Pneu PAC note the hollow tube protruding from the retangular box at the top of the cylinder (opposite the key). When the cylinder is turned on a painted

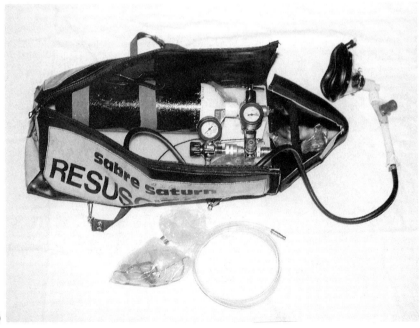

(a)

bar rises up inside the tube. The amount of painted bar seen through the small hole in the tube indicates the fraction of oxygen contained in the cylinder. Always use an oral airway when using the resuscitator function to facilitate a clear airway (the Pneu PAC has a warning noise to indicate if the airway is blocked). Which ever type of resuscitator your service uses, always ensure that you read the instruction manual carefully, this is the only way you will be fully conversant with it

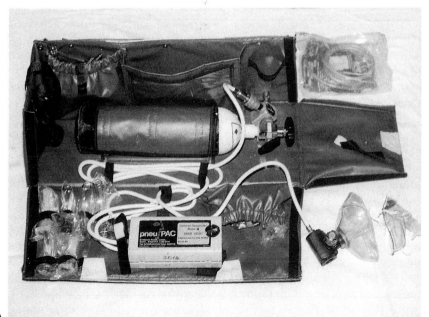

(b)

Appendix C

Driving Skills

Regional ambulance training schools run a two week driving course for ambulance personnel. This is based on the manual 'Roadcraft' which is used for the police driving courses. The ambulance course is thoroughly recommended by the author but the mechanics of driving do not fall within the scope of this book. We are concerned only with the attitude of a driver to his or her driving with a patient on board.

Very few people are prepared to accept criticism of their own driving standards although they often criticise freely the driving of others. The example can be quoted of a crew who regularly used the *same* criticism of each other's driving! What a pity they could not have experienced their own driving skills as a passenger.

There is a vast difference in stability and comfort between riding in the front of an ambulance and travelling in the rear saloon. The driver is sitting on a single seat facing the front, able to see what is happening and to anticipate braking and acceleration. The weight of the engine prevents the front from bouncing excessively. The patient in the rear saloon is either sitting sideways or is lying on a trolley (which feels unstable) facing the rear of the vehicle. He or she cannot anticipate the braking or accelerating and each provokes a reflex action within the patient's body. The rear of the vehicle is only carrying a fraction of its maximum load and consequently bounces over the bumps. The faster the ambulance is travelling (motorways excepted) the worse this is. The same applies to cornering. Whereas the driver can see the corner approaching and is prepared, the patient cannot and the movement again provokes reflex actions within the patient's body.

The difference is so marked that if an ambulance is driven the way a private car is driven, e.g. keeping up with traffic, pulling out quickly into gaps, cornering sharply and not reducing speed over bumpy roads, the patient and attendant will be given an uncomfortable ride even though it feels fine to the driver.

This uncomfortable ride is exacerbated by hard braking, rapid acceleration and fast cornering. Indeed Dr Snook of Bath, who has spent a great deal of time in connection with ambulance training, has stated that all these have a detrimental effect on the stretcher patient's internal organs. Much time and money has also been spent in trying to provide a reasonably priced floating stretcher so that the effects on the patient of both the driving and the road surface can be minimised.

It is obvious from this, therefore, that the way an ambulance is driven will have a considerable effect on any patient carried. A steady, smooth drive will ensure that the patient has a comfortable ride and complement the attendant's treatment, whereas, a thoughtless drive at normal speeds will cause discomfort and undo much of the attendant's work.

Yet a number of ambulance personnel drive an ambulance the same way irrespective of whether they have a patient on board or not. Some even drive more slowly when they are empty and then speed up when carrying a patient. This is totally wrong.

Smoothness is even more important if a fast ride is required. The system of car control which is taught at the regional training schools is completely compatible with this except that the driver must remember that with a patient on board, the first priority is a smooth ride and making progress is the second. Always drive for your patient and not for yourself.

Areas for Consideration

Speed

How comfortable the ambulance is at speed is directly related to the type of road surface and the nature of the road in relation to its environment. 60 mph will produce different results on a motorway than on an inner city road. Speed must vary depending on the state of the road surface. What is important is to drive at a speed which gives a comfortable ride and allows the attendant to work in the back. Even when a fast ride is required these criteria must apply. The driver should also keep an eye on the rear saloon so that if, for example, the patient begins to vomit, he or she can slow down without the attendant having to ask.

Acceleration

Always accelerate steadily with a patient on board. Depress the accelerator slowly until the desired speed is reached. Do not put the accelerator down hard, which produces rapid acceleration, and then ease off when the vehicle is travelling fast enough.

Braking

Braking should be smooth and progressive especially on vehicles with an assisted braking system where the pressure on the pedal does not need to be hard to slow the vehicle down. Judge the distance in which the vehicle is to be stopped, bearing in mind road conditions, and gradually increase the pressure on the pedal to produce a progressive slowing of the vehicle. Do not press the pedal hard to produce a rapid deceleration and then ease off to coast up to the stopping place. As the vehicle stops, try to ease off the pedal at the last minute to prevent the vehicle jerking back as it does so.

Cornering

The vehicle should be driven around a corner or bend using enough acceleration to keep the vehicle stable and prevent lateral pressures. This does not mean it has to be driven round fast. In town driving the speed of the vehicle should be gently reduced when approaching the corner so that it can then be driven equally as gently round it. Bends should be taken smoothly and again this may mean adjusting the speed on approach.

Conclusion

Drive the vehicle the way you would want it driven if you had a very sick patient in the back whom you were treating. It requires concentration, thought, forward vision and anticipation as well as a large amount of skill but is well worth the effort for the benefit of your patients.

Index